Hirschsprung's Disease

Solving The Puzzle

An Informational Resource Guide
for Parents & Medical Professionals

Nicole B. Murphy, Teacher (MST) & Mom

DISCLAIMER
This publication is not to be used for the diagnosis or treatment of
Hirschsprung's Disease. It is not a substitute for consultation with
licensed medical professionals. As new medical or scientific information
becomes available, recommended treatments may change. The reader
is advised to check with a physician before administering any drug
mentioned in this book. The author is not responsible for the content of
any web pages or publications referenced in this book.

COPYRIGHT NOTICE
*This book is intended for educational purposes. Illegal copying of this book
will only decrease the amount of money given towards Hirschsprung's
Disease research. A portion of the profits from this book will be donated to
The Hirschsprung's Gift Fund at Johns Hopkins School of Medicine Institute of
Genetic Medicine.*

"Guidelines for Caring for Your Ill Child," reprinted with permission from
www.babyheartspress.com.

To purchase a copy of this manual, please go to
www.hirschsprungsdiseasehelp.org.

DEDICATION

*This book is dedicated to my son Kellen. Without him,
this book would not have come to be. His fun-loving personality
kept me going on this project when I felt discouraged.
It is my hope that this book will answer some of the many questions
parents and medical staff may have about the rare disorder
called Hirschsprung's Disease.*

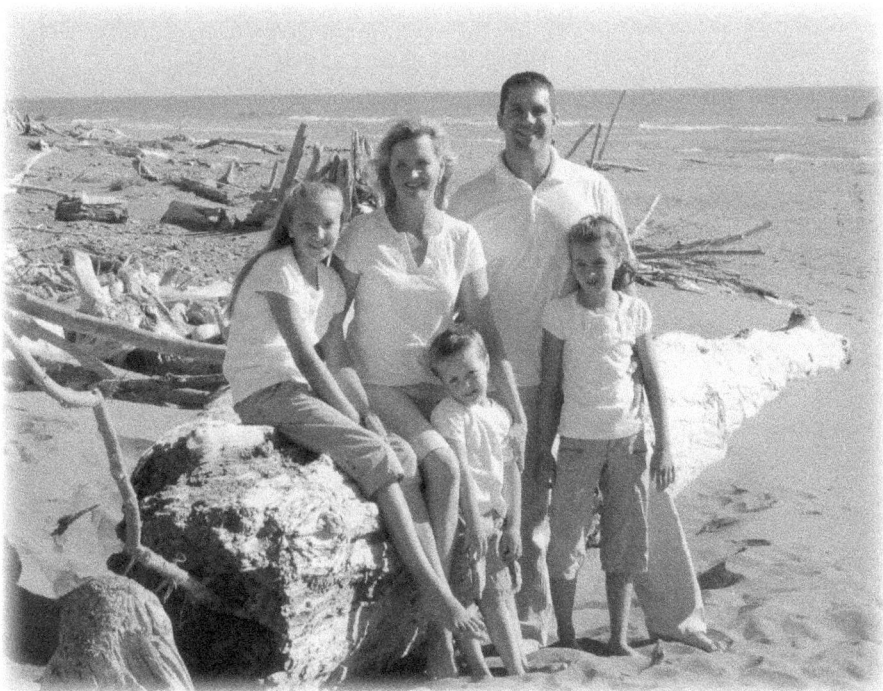

Clockwise from left: Jesslyn, Nicole, Bryan, Brooke and Kellen.

ACKNOWLEDGEMENTS

I would like to thank pediatric surgeons Dr. David Bliss and Dr. Tom Curran who performed Kellen's pull-through operations, Doctors Alan Merritt and Peter Boehm who first diagnosed Kellen, and Dr. Dale Svendsen who continues his care today. I would also like to thank all of the nurses who cared for Kellen throughout his illness (especially Kathy Gould, Michelle Stanley, and Barbara Wartell). Thanks also to Monica Forte who wrote the Stoma, TPN, and Mickey button care sections, and my mother and Mackenzie Edlund for their drawings.

I would especially like to thank geneticist Julie Albertus Muskett, formerly of Johns Hopkins Medical School, for her help with the genetics section of the manual, Shelly Blumberg for editing the book, Carol White for her marketing help and Anita Jones for the typesetting. A special thanks goes to Dr. Tom Curran and Dr. Marc Levitt for their help in this latest revision. I am extremely grateful to all of my friends for all of their input and guidance. Finally, many thanks to my professor Dr. Phil Hoffman for encouraging me to write the book in the first place.

My special appreciation goes to my daughters Brooke and Jesslyn, my son Kellen, and my husband Bryan for their patience with me during the six years it took me to write this book.

CONTENTS

Introduction

Prior to the birth of my children, I taught science and health for ten years. I loved teaching but chose to stay at home after the birth of my second child Brooke. Four years later, we had our son Kellen.

It turned out that Kellen was born with Hirschsprung's Disease, a rare disorder of the colon. During this time, I was renewing my teaching license and had to take an independent research course in science or health through our local college. I was required to write three large term papers on a topic in my field: so naturally, I chose Hirschsprung's Disease (The actual genetic abbreviation is HSCR, however, I will refer to Hirschsprung's Disease as HD throughout the manual).

When Kellen was first diagnosed, I was handed a little brochure on Hirschsprung's Disease. While it had basic information in it about the disease, I wanted to know more. After one year of writing and research, I completed my three term papers. At the urging of my professor, I decided to publish what I had learned for other parents dealing with HD. Three years later, the book has finally come to fruition. It is my hope that what I have learned through my experiences will help others to better understand this complex and frightening disease.

KELLEN'S STORY

ON NOVEMBER FOURTH, 2003, we had our baby boy Kellen Baxter Murphy. Weighing in at 8 lbs. 12 oz, he was a big, chubby, healthy looking boy. Kellen looked perfect on the outside yet little did we know that on the inside, he was not well. A few hours after he was born, I tried nursing Kellen but he had no interest at all. I figured that he was just still tired from labor so I let him rest for a while. Later that day, I tried again and still no luck. No one seemed too worried, so I just rested with him by my side.

The next morning, we tried nursing again. This time, I had the lactation nurse come in to help me. While the nurse was in there, Kellen spit up a little bit of greenish/yellowish looking liquid onto the sheets of my bed. She said, "Something is not right with this baby, he doesn't want to eat." So we put him back into the bassinet and she did a thorough exam. Right away, she noticed that Kellen was breathing faster than normal. She also noticed that his abdomen was distended and made a note that he had not had his first stool (*meconium*) yet.

St. Charles NICU

When the nurse told me that they needed to take Kellen to the NICU (neonatal intensive care unit) and run some tests on him, my heart just sank. I called my husband and told him the bad news.

When we went in later to see him, he had a tube down his nose and an IV in his head. It was very disturbing to see him this way. After the preliminary tests, we were sent down to radiology for an upper GI. The radiologist gave Kellen a "drink" through his tube of a Gastrografin, which would show any blockage in the intestine. It was then that the technicians found the meconium plug. At this point, the doctors thought the plug could be caused by gestational diabetes or Cystic Fibrosis. We were hoping that it would be the former.

That night, we came home from the hospital without our baby. I remember going into Kellen's bedroom and looking at the crib. I just broke down in tears. I was so worried about Kellen that I didn't sleep a wink that night. I prayed that he would not have Cystic Fibrosis and fortunately, this was not the case.

I arrived at the hospital at 8:00am Friday morning. I walked into the NICU and saw my baby laying there with so many tubes in him. As I was sitting beside Kellen, Dr. Boehm, a pediatrician at Central Oregon Pediatrics, came to sit beside me and said, "Nicole, the plot thickens." I said, "What do you mean?" He then proceeded to tell me that they thought my baby had a rare disorder called Hirschsprung's Disease. I said, "Hirsch what?" I had never heard of Hirschsprung's Disease.

Dr. Boehm then led me over to the x-ray area and Dr. Merritt, our local neonatologist, showed me the point at which the colon was rather large on the x-rays. He said that the width of the colon should be the same width as the spine. A section of Kellen's colon was much larger and almost twice as wide and the area below the large part of the colon appeared to be atrophied.

Dr. Boehm said, "unfortunately, we cannot handle this here." "This disease is fixable with an operation but you are going to need to go for an airplane ride to Emanuel Children's Hospital in Portland." I felt like I had been hit by a ton of bricks. Not five minutes ago, I thought everything was going to be just fine.

I called to inform my husband Bryan that we would be getting on the Airlife plane in about 30 minutes. He would have to meet us over in Portland. Usually I am afraid to fly but I just couldn't leave my baby. I didn't want to be anywhere but on that plane with Kellen.

Airlife

The Airlife team came in and prepped us for transport. I was still in shock. Bryan brought me a bag of clothes and my breast pump and was going to drive over and meet us. They would only let one of us go on the airplane because of the weight restrictions. My mother-in-law stayed with my older two girls, which was a relief to both of us.

We were taken by ambulance to the Bend Airport. Kellen was in an incubator with high-tech monitors all around him. The Airlife Plane we boarded was one of the new Turbo Single Prop Airplanes and the pilot was retired from the Air Force. It was such a smooth flight that Kellen slept the whole way to Portland, even during the landing. The nurse and the respiratory therapist monitored his vital signs during the flight. I felt like I was having a bad dream.

Arriving at Emanuel

Once we landed in Portland, we were then taken by another ambulance to Emanuel Children's Hospital. There, some very nice nurses greeted us. I remember thinking how much larger this NICU was compared to the NICU in Bend. There were only five babies at St. Charles compared to around 100 or more at Emanuel.

A curtain separated each bed. There were rows upon rows of them. Kellen was put in the ducky area right next to a nice big room with a bathroom and shower. This room would be my home for the next few weeks.

Meeting the doctors and nurses

Dr. Tom Curran, a pediatric surgeon and his resident came in later that day and took a biopsy of Kellen's colon. This was done to see if he had the proper nerve cells in the colon lining. These nerves help to move digested food through the body. If the cells were absent, Kellen would need surgery. If there were cells there, Hirschsprung's Disease could be ruled out. Later that day, the biopsy results came back positive for HD. Dr. Curran explained that Kellen lacked nerve cells in about 6 inches of his colon and that he would be performing an operation called a pull-through. He showed us diagrams and explained what he would be doing.

Because Kellen was so chubby, the nurses had a hard time finding veins for IV's. They finally found one that worked in his head but they told us it might not hold long. The nurses were unsuccessful at putting a *PICC line* (a longer lasting IV) in also. Luckily, Dr. Curran was able to move Kellen up on his surgery schedule.

The Ronald McDonald House

Bryan and I had a really nice room at The Ronald McDonald House but I only stayed there the first night. I couldn't bear to leave Kellen after that. I sat by his bed all day and at night I usually slept in a recliner so I could watch the monitors. Except for one time, I left only to eat or go to the bathroom. I became Kellen's primary care person. The nurses taught me how to do a lot of things.

Baptism and preparing for surgery

One of the hardest parts of the ordeal was getting Kellen ready for the surgery. He was so hungry because he hadn't had anything in six days. Now that his stomach had been emptied of the bile, he was starting to feel hungry. I couldn't feed him because his intestines had to be cleaned out for the surgery. The nurses allowed him to have sugar water on his pacifier to help with the hunger pains. I can't imagine how hungry he must have been. I pumped milk every two hours around the clock to keep my milk supply going. I wanted Kellen to have breast milk because it is so much easier to digest than formula. This would be very important for him in the future.

My sister Shannon called her priest Father Dan to come to Emanuel and baptize Kellen. I didn't want to admit it, but anytime a child goes in for surgery, there are risks involved. Bryan and I were just sick to our stomachs but tried to put on a happy face for the occasion. Father Dan did a wonderful job. We did feel some relief that Kellen would be in heaven if something went wrong.

The night before surgery, the night nurse flushed out Kellen's system with a liquid called "Go Lightly." It got rid of all that was left in his intestines. When I returned the next morning she told me Kellen's blood pressure went way up because he had a hard time passing the Go Lightly. In hindsight, an irrigation tube would have helped him pass the contrast medium. I never left his side after that.

Operation day

Kellen's operation was scheduled for Tuesday, November 11th at 5:00 p.m. We went down to the operating room and said goodbye to Kellen. Then, the nurse showed us the waiting room. There were only a few people in there. Bryan and I had brought along a deck of cards. We thought that if we played Rummy, it would keep our minds off of the surgery. It felt like time moved in slow motion. We had never felt so much stress and worry in our lives.

Kellen's operation ended up taking six hours because the surgeon had to send the biopsies down to the lab for the technician to read. The doctor has to be sure that entire diseased portion of the intestine is removed. When the technician begins to see the nerve cells in the intestinal wall biopsies, the surgeon can proceed with the operation.

After what seemed like an eternity, Dr. Curran came into the waiting room and told us all went well. It was as if a huge weight was lifted off of our shoulders. I didn't realize however, that the hardest part was yet to come.

Post-op

When they brought Kellen out of the Operating Room, we were shocked at what we saw. He was bloated from all of the fluids they had given him and he was on a respirator. He didn't look like our baby boy.

The time came to remove the respirator. A team of nurses and doctors stood around him. I had a gut feeling that he wasn't ready to breathe on his own yet. As it turned out, I was right. When they removed the breathing tube, Kellen turned bright blue! It was so scary. They had to re-intubate him on the spot. Kellen was removed from the respirator 24 hours later with no problems.

Kellen had some problems with pain after the surgery. The morphine would cause him to stop breathing. It was a very stressful time. We watched his chest rise and fall for two days straight. Finally, the nurses gave him an analgesic called Toradol that worked wonderfully. They had to make sure that he had healed enough inside because of the possibility of internal bleeding. Some analgesics, like aspirin and Toradol, can cause bleeding.

In the next week, Kellen had to learn to drink the milk I had saved for him. I think there were at least 50 bottles in the freezer. He caught on really fast and guzzled every last drop. Kellen quickly began to gain weight and poop on his own. I never thought I would be so excited about a poop! The nurses said that once he learned to do these things, we could go home. We left the hospital on November 18th, 2003.

Going home

It was such a relief to finally have our baby home. We had to return in a week to meet with Dr. Curran so he could make sure that everything was going well. Kellen seemed to be doing okay with the pooping but not as well as we would have hoped. He still didn't go as often as my two girls did but we just figured that would be normal for him.

Bryan and I drove Kellen over for his first post-op check up. In order to check the *anastomosis* (the point where the healthy colon is sewn to the rectum), Dr. Curran had to put on a glove and insert his finger into Kellen's anus. When he did this a large amount of diarrhea came out, and Kellen cried really hard. Dr. Curran then showed us how to do a dilatation. He gently put the metal rod into Kellen's anus and even greener smelly poop came out. He told us that we would have to do this procedure twice a day. As the weeks went on, we would be required to use a rod with a larger circumference until the sutured portion was stretched to the required width. It was not a pleasant thing to have to do to a baby. The ride home was quiet as we adjusted to the realization that this would be part of our daily routine for the next few months.

Back to Emanuel

As the days went by, Kellen pooped less and less and we were beginning to get worried about him. Kellen just didn't look good to me and he had stopped pooping altogether. He was really pale and lethargic.

We knew something wasn't right so I immediately called the surgeon's office and spoke with Dr. Bliss, Dr. Curran's partner. After I explained Kellen's symptoms, he told me to get into my car and drive him to Emanuel in Portland immediately. This was about a three-hour drive from where we lived. He told me that he had babies die of something called *enterocolitis* (a serious illness caused by inflammation and infection of the colon) because their parents didn't listen and get help for their child. Luckily, my dad was in town so he drove us over and we went directly to the hospital. This time, we were admitted into the Pediatric Unit.

The doctors ordered an x-ray first to be sure there was no blockage. After the x-ray came back normally, they performed another upper GI to clean out his gut. He did some beautiful pooping after that, but only for a short time. The doctors also did a blood test to rule out enterocolitis. We were released again and went home but I still felt that something was wrong.

Home again

For about a month, Bryan and I continued to do the dilatations and the irrigations on a daily basis. Each week, we would drive to the hospital for Kellen's checkup. As the weeks progressed, the dilatation rods got bigger and bigger and we had to go fewer and fewer times to see the doctor. Kellen still wasn't pooping very well and he was still crying during the dilatations.

To Emanuel once again

I can't remember the details of our next visit to Emanuel, but I do remember it was around Thanksgiving. Once again, Kellen was not pooping well and the doctors wanted to test him for enterocolitis.

Everything checked out all right and the surgeons told us to just keep doing the irrigations and dilatations until he started pooping on his own. Sometimes, it takes the anal sphincter awhile to relax after a pull-through operation so many babies have to have these procedures done to them for a few months.

The next month was a struggle. Kellen was getting bigger and stronger and it was harder to do the "procedure" as Bryan and I called it. It took both of us to do it properly. It must have really hurt him because he cried really hard every time. We felt horrible doing this to him every day but we knew it was necessary.

More vomiting

It was two days before Christmas when he became ill again. I noticed that again he looked very pale and was acting lethargic. When I tried to nurse him, he threw up all over me. Immediately, I called my pediatrician and they told me to come in. One of Kellen's doctors at Central Oregon Pediatrics examined him and said he really wasn't sick enough to admit to the hospital. He told me to go home and try to nurse him again. If he threw up another time, we could be admitted to the hospital. There was no abdominal distention or fever present and we were both confused about the cause of vomiting.

I went back home and tried feeding him again and sure enough, he threw up all over me. Because it is a smaller hospital, the pediatric unit at St. Charles consists of only a few rooms. Kellen was the only baby there that day. He continued to throw up throughout the day and we became extremely worried about him. Bryan and I knew we had a very sick baby so we asked to be airlifted to Emanuel. The doctor agreed with our decision because his surgeons were there and could evaluate him.

Airlife ride #2

Kellen and I were becoming frequent flyers on the Air Life plane. After we were admitted to the Pediatric Unit, tests were run and everything came back looking fine. Kellen and I spent Christmas in the hospital that year. Bryan stayed home with the girls and had help from his mother and stepfather. Thank goodness for family! I really missed my girls but I knew I had to be with the baby. This time, Kellen and I hitched a ride home to Bend with my father-in-law and his fiancé. For a short time after this hospital stay, Kellen had good bowel movements.

More procedures

Over the next few months, Bryan and I continued to do the "procedure." We made our monthly trips over to Portland to see Dr. Curran. Kellen was still having a lot of pain during the dilations.

According to Dr. Curran, he should have been getting more used to them by now. As time went on, he cried harder and harder during the procedure and he was getting stronger and stronger. We had to hold him down really hard—I felt like I was torturing my baby.

One particular day after we had done the procedure, Kellen started bleeding. I called Dr. Curran and he told me I had to go back to doing the dilations twice a day or the scar tissue (*stricture*) would close down on him. The bleeding showed that the anastomosis had not healed properly and there could be a lack of blood supply to the area. The tissue then just basically died. Dr. Curran said this was causing a mechanical problem in the intestine and that he would have to re-do the operation. Bryan and I were just devastated.

Operation #2

Kellen's second surgery was scheduled for April ninth, which was Good Friday. We would again be in the hospital over a holiday weekend. This time it was Easter. Bryan and I had been giving him up to five irrigations a day because he could not get rid of the gas or feces in his colon. The stricture had really closed down on him. We were relieved to have him "fixed" so that he could have a normal life but we were also really scared to have him go through another operation. Dr. Curran wanted to wait until Kellen was at least five months old before he re-did the pull-through.

We went through the same routine again but this time, when they checked his blood pressure, it was really low. He had gotten dehydrated from all of the enemas I had been giving him. I felt relieved that we were in the hospital and he could be put on an IV. This time, when we walked with him down to surgery, I cried the whole way. I just had a big pit in my stomach. Bryan felt really nervous about it also. We knew he was in great hands but it was still really hard to let him go.

I went down to the Chapel and said a lot of prayers. I begged God to let him get through the surgery okay. That moment was a major turning point in my life. I felt much calmer afterwards and went back up to Kellen's room to wait.

A funny clown came in and did some magic tricks for us. He was really good and kept our minds off of the surgery for a while. At one point, I put my running shoes on and ran up and down the stairs because I needed some sort of outlet from all of the stress. With about an hour left of the surgery, Bryan and I went down to the OR waiting area.

After six hours, Dr. Curran came out and told us that everything went really well. His associate, Dr. David Bliss, assisted him this time. They had removed the scar tissue and because Kellen's colon was so much larger now, we wouldn't have to do the dilations after surgery. We felt like jumping for joy! Kellen and I stayed in the hospital while he recovered for three more days. He eventually started having bowel movements and when he could eat normally, we got to go home.

Home at last

Bryan and I still had to do the irrigations for a while until Kellen learned how to relax his anal sphincter muscle. We did the irrigations for two months until he started to go on his own. It has been nearly seven years since his second pull-through and five years ago that we were able to quit doing the irrigations.

Looking back, I have to say that those three years were the scariest of my life. The worst part was not knowing what to do for Kellen most of the time. The uncertainty of what was causing Kellen to be so sick was terrible. We were admitted to our local ER many times because Kellen was just not doing well. Tests would be run and the results would show nothing. The doctors and I were so confused.

Looking back, I can see that he had chronic mild to moderate bouts of enterocolitis caused by a stricture. At the time, I thought that in order to have enterocolitis, bacteria had to show up in the blood work. After researching enterocolitis further, I discovered that this is not the case. Children do not have to have bacterial enterocolitis but can have HAEC (Hirschsprung Associated Enterocolitis) after a pull-through operation.

Dr. Curran suggested that the mechanical problem was causing the enterocolitis and once the scar tissue was removed and the operation was redone, the bouts of enterocolitis would decrease significantly. Fortunately for us, he was right. After the second operation, Kellen improved notably and we could start living our lives again. I have never had such a scary experience in my life. We are so blessed that today he is a happy, healthy, seven-year-old little boy.

WHAT IS HIRSCHSPRUNG'S DISEASE?

HIRSCHSPRUNG'S (HURSH-SPRUNGZ) DISEASE (HD) is a disease affecting the large intestine, otherwise known as the colon. Some other names for Hirschsprung's Disease are *Congenital Megacolon and Colonic Aganglionosis* (meaning without nerve cells). It is a congenital disease, which means a person is born with it. Hirschsprung's Disease also has hereditary components and could be passed on from parent to child. It is a rare disease that affects one in 5,000 live births. HD occurs four times more often in boys than in girls (NIDDK, 2003).

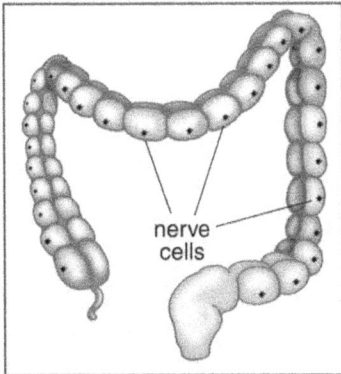

Figure 1. No Hirschsprung's Disease
Nerve cells found throughout
the small intestine and colon.

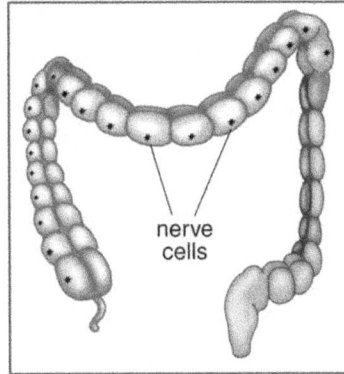

Figure 2. Hirschsprung's Disease
Nerve cells are missing from
the small intestine and colon.

Images reproduced with permission from the National Institute of
Diabetes and Digestive and Kidney Diseases, National Institute of Health, 2010.

Hirschsprung's Disease occurs when nerve cells are absent in the intestinal wall. Nerve cells act as messengers that carry electrical impulses through the body. In Hirschsprung's Disease, these cells (otherwise called *ganglion* cells) are absent making complete digestion and elimination of feces difficult or impossible. The lack of nerve cells in part of the intestine interrupts the electrical signals from the brain and prevents *peristalsis* (contractions of muscles that propel feces through intestines) from occurring (see Figures 1 and 2).

THE HISTORY OF HIRSCHSPRUNG'S DISEASE

ANATOMIST FREDERICK RUYSCH, who observed an intestinal obstruction in a deceased five-year-old girl, first described Hirschsprung's Disease in the 17th century. He wrote about an "enormous dilatation of the colon." (Ruysch, F., 1691). The Danish physician Harald Hirschsprung of Copenhagen, Denmark, after whom the disease was named, presented the first clinical description of Hirschsprung's Disease at the Berlin Society of Pediatrics in 1886 (See Figure 3).

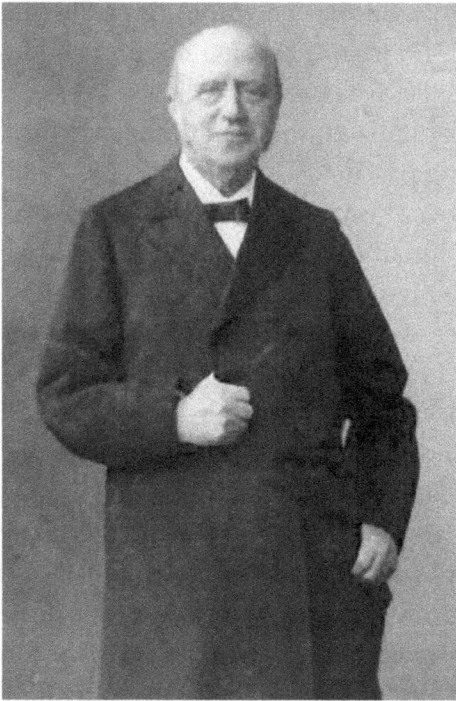

Figure 3. Dr. Harald Hirschsprung
Image reprinted with permission from Wikimedia Commons, 2011.

At the Berlin Congress for Children's Diseases, Hirschsprung gave a lecture about what would eventually become "his" disease. Dr. Hirschsprung discovered that the two infants he spoke about had died from constipation associated with an increase in size of the colon (Hirschsprung, 1888).

In 1901, Tittel saw that an absence of *ganglion* (nerve) cells in the colon toward the rectum was the actual cause of Hirschsprung's. Theodore Ehrenpries, in 1946, discovered that the colon became enlarged and distended because of an obstruction caused by the lack of ganglion cells in the intestinal wall. However, it wasn't until 1948 that surgeon Ovar Swenson performed the first successful *pull-through* operation (Swenson & Bill, (1948).

Joseph Vincent Murphy Jr. was the first patient to undergo a pull-through operation. He spent the first three years of his life in the hospital and his family said that he would have died had it not been for Dr. Swenson. In 1946, Joseph became the first child to survive a pull-through operation. He was unable to play sports as a child because he was frequently hospitalized, so his father taught him how to sail. This became his life-long passion.

Mr. Murphy went on to enlist in the Navy, served for two years, and later built and maintained naval ships. Mr. Murphy lived a long, happy, and productive life, thanks to the groundbreaking operation known as the Swenson pull-through. This procedure is now the most common treatment for Hirschsprung's Disease.

Because physicians are now more aware of HD, more babies are being diagnosed shortly after birth. They are therefore less likely to suffer from *enterocolitis* (an infection of the colon), infection, and ruptured colon as many have before them. In 1954, the mortality rate among newborns with HD was 70%. In 1992 the rate fell to six percent and in 2000 it fell again to one percent (American Pediatric Association (APA), 2000). If HD is left untreated, stool can fill up in the large intestine causing infection, bursting of the colon and even death. Before operations for HD became available, many babies died of Hirschsprung's Disease.

SYMPTOMS OF HIRSCHSPRUNG'S DISEASE

USUALLY, SYMPTOMS OF HD begin just a few days after birth. It is estimated that 80% of children with HD show symptoms in the first six weeks of life (Schneider Children's Hospital, 2006). The main symptom of HD in infants is the inability to pass the *meconium* (first stool) within the first 24 to 48 hours of life (see Figure 4).

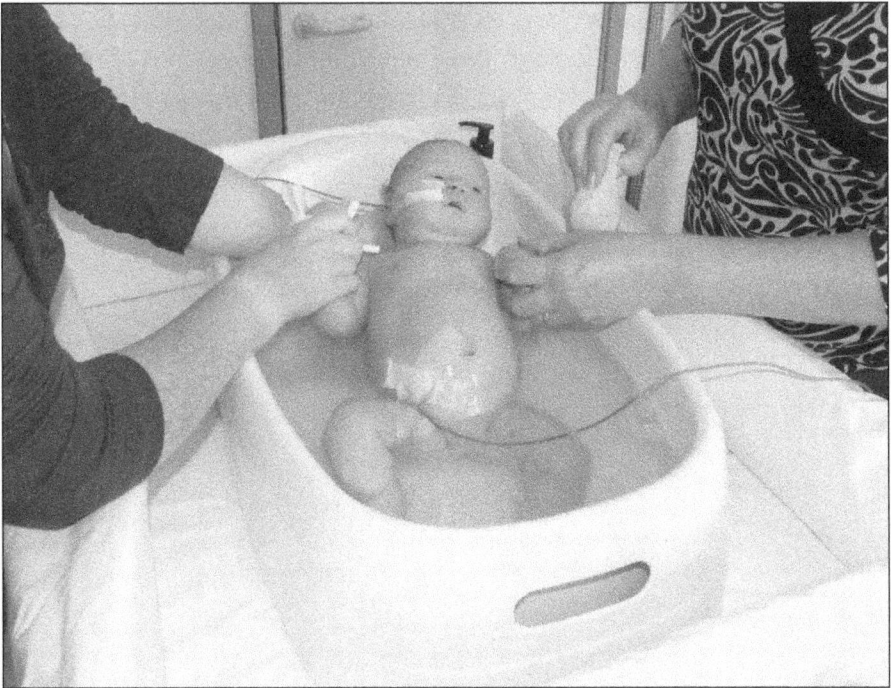

Figure 4. Abdominal distention in newborn baby.
Image reprinted with permission from Hirschsprungshelp@yahoo.com, 2009.

The main symptoms of Hirschsprung's Disease are:
- Vomiting of bile
- Abdominal *distention* (bloating)
- Chronic constipation
- Diarrhea
- Enterocolitis (inflammation of the small intestine and colon)

In some cases, however, people don't develop symptoms until childhood or adulthood. These people usually have a short segment of intestine that lacks normal nerve cells. In older children, there is almost always a history of poor bowel movements.

Usually, these children have protruding abdomens, may pass small watery stools, have diarrhea, lack of appetite and show signs of fatigue. They can also have constipation, *anemia* (a shortage of red blood cells) from lost blood in the stool, malnutrition, and can suffer from delayed growth. Advanced disease can cause *sepsis* (a life-threatening bloodborne infection).

HIRSCHSPRUNG'S DISEASE
AND THE DIGESTIVE SYSTEM

THE DIGESTIVE SYSTEM is a muscular tube that extends from the mouth to the anus. The digestive system includes the mouth, teeth, tongue, esophagus, stomach, small intestine, large intestine, rectum and anal canal. It measures about 6-9 meters long when fully extended. The pancreas and liver are also an integral part of the digestive system (see Figure 5).

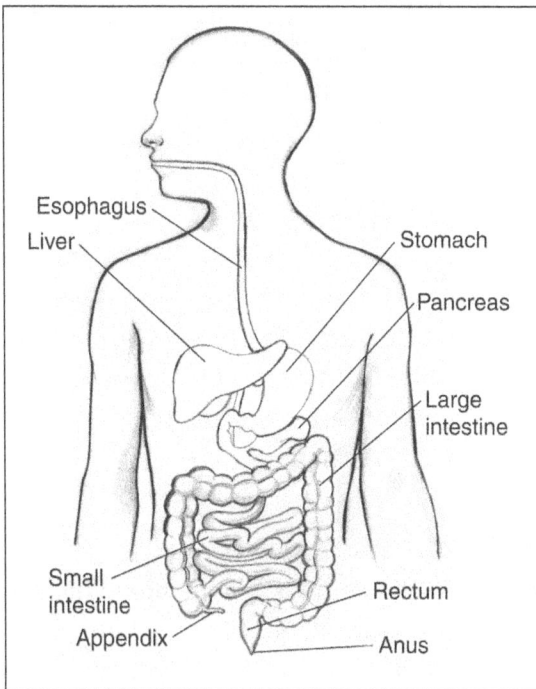

Figure 5. The digestive system

Image reprinted with permission from the National Institute of
Diabetes and Digestive and Kidney Diseases, National Institute of Health, 2010.

Small intestine

The stomach empties into the small intestine, the longest part of the digestive tract. It measures about 18 feet long. The small intestine absorbs nutrients from the food we eat. The main parts of the small intestine are the *duodenum* (at the base of the stomach), the *jejunum* (the next six to seven feet of intestine), and the *ileum* (the remaining ten or so feet of intestine).

Pancreas and liver

The pancreas and liver aid in the breakdown of nutrients in the small intestine. The pancreas secretes digestive enzymes that break down carbohydrates, proteins, and fats (*lipids*). Bile from the liver helps in the digestion of fats. Most digestion occurs in the small intestine as well as absorption of nutrients. In rare cases, part of the small intestine is affected by Hirschsprung's Disease causing more nutritional problems in the child.

Large intestine

The large intestine is about five feet long. It is also known as the colon (see Figure 6). The four main parts of the colon are the ascending colon, the transverse colon, the descending colon, and the sigmoid colon. No significant digestion occurs in the large intestine. The main purpose of the colon is to absorb sodium, chloride, and water. Hirschsprung's Disease usually occurs in this area, so patients with HD have to be careful of dehydration after the operation.

Rectum and anal canal

Located below the sigmoid colon is the rectum, which is comprised of muscles that help to move the stool out of the body (see Figure 6). The internal and external sphincter muscles surround the anal canal. The internal sphincter muscles are involuntary, meaning a person cannot control them. The external sphincter muscles are voluntary, meaning a person normally can control their bowel movements.

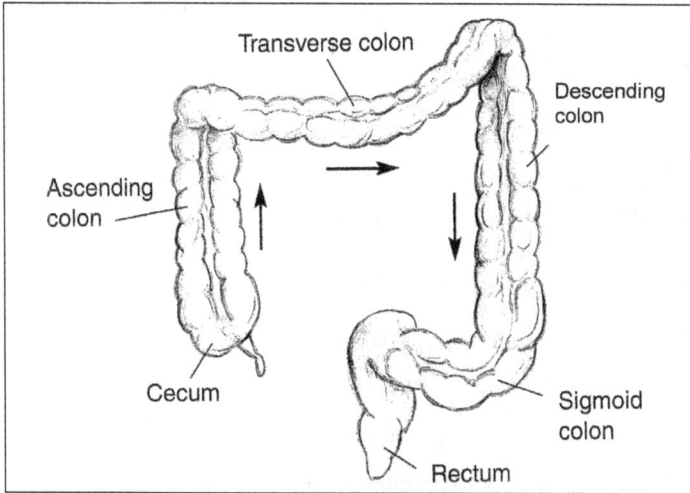

Figure 6. The colon.
Image reprinted with permission from The National Institute of
Diabetes and Digestive and Kidney Diseases, National Institute of Health, 2010.

Peristalsis

Peristalsis is the rhythmic contraction or squeezing of muscles surrounding the intestine that propels material through the gut so it can be digested and eventually eliminated (see Figure 7). Without the nerve cells in the segment of colon affected by HD, the diseased portion cannot relax and move the bowel contents through the intestinal tract. So, it is almost like the intestine stalls in that area and cannot help to push the stool through.

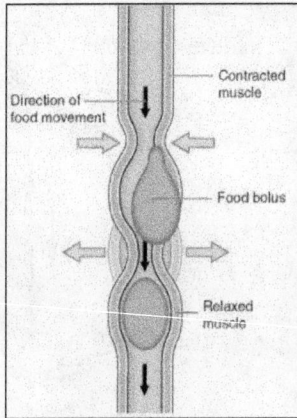

Figure 7. Peristalsis

Image reprinted with permission from the Medical-Dictionary. Thefreedictionary.com, 2010.

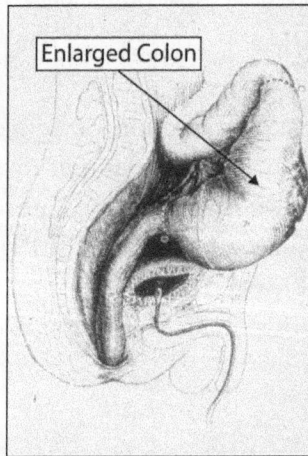

Figure 8. Classical megacolon.

Image reprinted with permission from Wikimedia Commons, 2011.

This causes the intestine to become partially or completely blocked, resulting in the upper portion of the colon expanding to a much larger than normal size, thus the term "Megacolon" (see Figure 8). It is estimated that HD causes 20% of intestinal obstructions in newborns (Children's Medical Encyclopedia, 2006).

HIRSCHSPRUNG'S DISEASE
AND THE NERVOUS SYSTEM

The central nervous system (CNS) consists of the brain and the spinal cord (see Figure 9). It is completely covered by bony structures — the brain in the skull and the spinal cord in the spinal column. The CNS is the control center of the nervous system and is located in the center of our body. It receives electrical messages from the other divisions of the nervous system and responds to them.

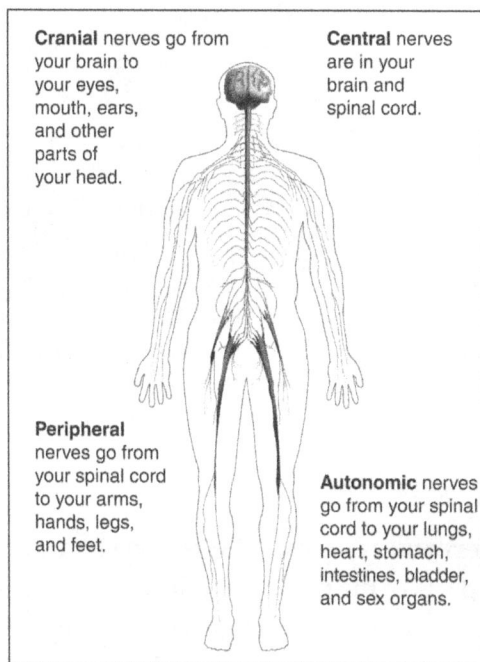

Cranial nerves go from your brain to your eyes, mouth, ears, and other parts of your head.

Central nerves are in your brain and spinal cord.

Peripheral nerves go from your spinal cord to your arms, hands, legs, and feet.

Autonomic nerves go from your spinal cord to your lungs, heart, stomach, intestines, bladder, and sex organs.

Figure 9. The Central Nervous System

Image reprinted with permission from The National Institute of Diabetes and Digestive and Kidney Diseases, National Institute of Health, 2010.

Sensory nerves collect input from the outside world and send it to the brain. The brain then sends electrical impulses through the motor nerves to the muscles and glands eliciting a response (see Figure 10). These messages can be relayed to and from various parts of the body at around the speed of light. The CNS is like a big computer while the other parts of the nervous system are like the various programs in the computer—all communicating with one another at various times when necessary.

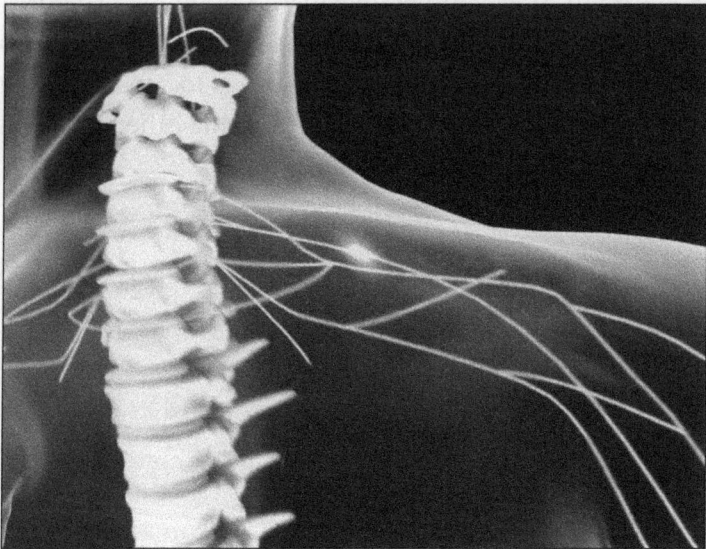

Figure 10. Electrical signal traveling along the nerve fiber
from the brain and spinal cord (CNS), to the outlying nerves (PNS).
Image reprinted with permission from Purdu Pharma L. P. © 2002

Peripheral nervous system

The peripheral nervous system (PNS) is a system of nerves that connect the outlying parts of the body with the central nervous system (see Figure 9). The PNS includes all of the nerves in the body except for the brain and spinal cord and is not covered by bony structures (skull & spinal column).

There are two main branches of the peripheral nervous system. The *afferent division* carries electrical impulses to the CNS from receptors in the skin and around the joints and the *efferent division*, which is further divided into three groups.

1. *The somatic nervous system or the voluntary nervous system.*

The motor functions in this system may be consciously controlled. The somatic motor nerves carry impulses from the CNS to the skeletal muscles. Examples of the skeletal muscles are the pectorals, glutes, biceps etc. The individual can largely control contractions of these muscles.

2. *The autonomic nervous system (ANS) or the involuntary nervous system.*

The motor functions of these muscles cannot be consciously controlled and are reflexive in nature. During emergencies that cause stress, the ANS allows us to take flight or fight, depending on what is endangering us. This is called the "fight or flight" response. In non-emergencies, the ANS allows us to "rest and digest." The ANS can further be divided into the sympathetic and parasympathetic divisions (see Figure 11).

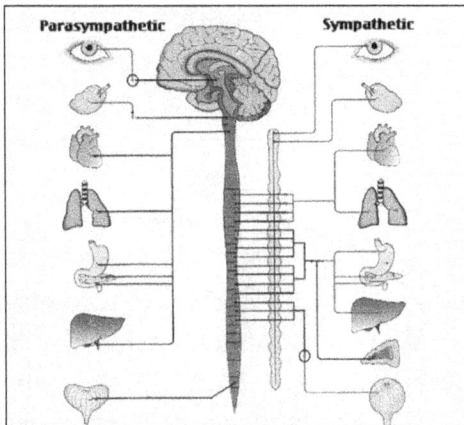

Figure 11. The autonomic nervous system. The ANS regulates the muscles in and around the skin, blood vessels, eyes, stomach, intestines, bladder and the heart.

Image reprinted with permission from users.rcn.com, 2010

A. Sympathetic nervous system. The nerves in this system are largely located in the spinal cord area from the neck down and then branch out to various organs in the body. Stimulation from this system causes the intestines to slow production.

B. Parasympathetic nervous system. The nerves in this system are largely located in the top and bottom portion of the spinal column and then branch out to organs and glands in that area. Stimulation from this system causes the intestines to speed up production.

3. Enteric nervous system (ENS).

The digestive system contains its own local nervous system called the ENS and is connected to the CNS via the vagus nerve. The ENS is a division of the autonomic nervous system (see Figure 12). Many scientists have called it "the second brain" because it is so complex (100 million nerves) and regulates so many activities in the gut (Wood, 2005). Basically, the ENS is responsible for keeping the intestines clean and protecting the body from external threats.

When the brain signals danger in the body, it tells the mast cells (cells found in the lining of the small intestine and/or colon that release chemicals in response to injury or inflammation) to liberate the chemicals heparin and histamine. These chemicals cause an inflammatory response inside the small intestine, attracting immune cells from the bloodstream into the area. Now, the body is prepared to deal with trauma, which can introduce infectious material into the colon (NSF, 2005).

Nervousness or fear can cause a person to have an upset stomach and diarrhea—an ENS response. When bacteria or other dangerous pathogens are found in the gut, a vomiting response may occur to "clean" out the intestines, all thanks to the ENS.

Another interesting aspect of the ENS is that it is trainable. During surgery for Hirschsprung's Disease, part of the colon is removed and the healthy parts are re-attached. The new piece of plumbing knows nothing about "pooping," yet it "learns" to perform this function within about 18 months. This tells scientists that the nerves have "learned" a new job (Wood, 2005).

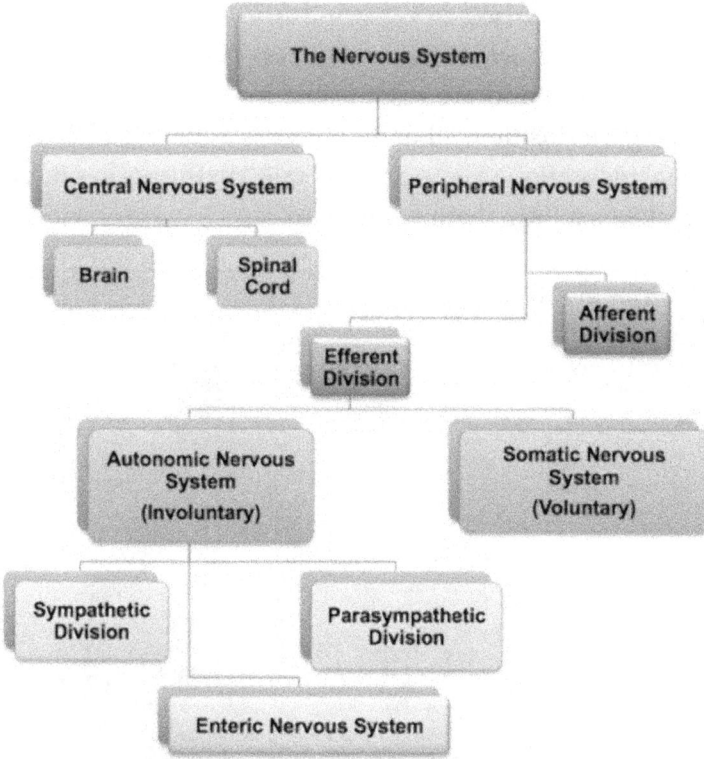

Figure 12. Map of the nervous system
Map created by Nicole Murphy, © 2010.

This system can and does function independently but also communicates with the central nervous system via the parasympathetic and sympathetic nerve fibers. The two main components of the enteric nervous system are two *plexuses* (networks) of neurons called the myenteric plexus and the submucosal plexus (see Figure 13). Both plexuses are embedded in the wall of the digestive tract and extend from the esophagus to the anus.

A. *The myenteric (Auerbach's) plexus.* These nerves are located between the longitudinal and circular layers of the muscle in the tunica muscularis and control digestive tract motility or peristalsis (wave-like motion of the gut). One of the criteria for diagnosis of HD is the absence of the ganglion cells in the myenteric and submucosal plexuses.

B. *The submucosal (Meissner's) plexus.* These nerves are located in the submucosa and are responsible for sensing the environment in the *lumen* (inside wall of the intestine) and regulating gastrointestinal blood flow. These nerves "talk" to the nerves in the myenteric plexus telling them what to do.

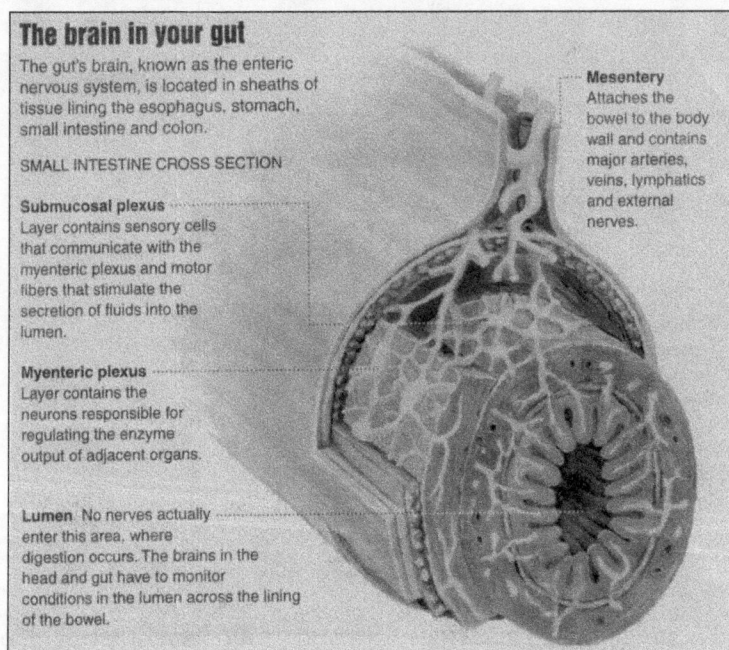

Figure 13. "The Brain in Your Gut."

Image reprinted with permission from *The Bulletin*, Friday, September 30th, 2005. "The Brain in your Gut," Dr. Michael D. Gershon, Columbia University (2005). The New York Times Service.

Neurons

The neuron, or nerve cell, is the basic unit of the nervous system. The main components of a nerve cell or neuron are the *dendrites* (branches of the cell body) and the *axon* (the nerve fibers). The dendrites are the receptive portion of the nerve cell where the electrical signals begin. The axon is the conductive portion of the neuron that transmits electrical signals. These electrical impulses then travel down the axon to another nerve or to the organs, muscles and glands (*effector* organs) relaying important information (see Figure 14).

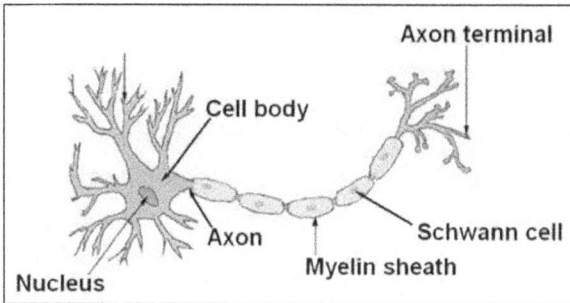

Figure 14. The nerve cell.
Image reprinted with permission from www.topnewin/files/nerve-cell, 2010

Neurotransmitters

The nerve cells do not directly touch one another but have a space between them called a synapse. A chemical called a neurotransmitter carries these signals across the synapse to either another nerve cell or organs (see Figure 15). There are many types of neurotransmitters in the body and each has a specific job.

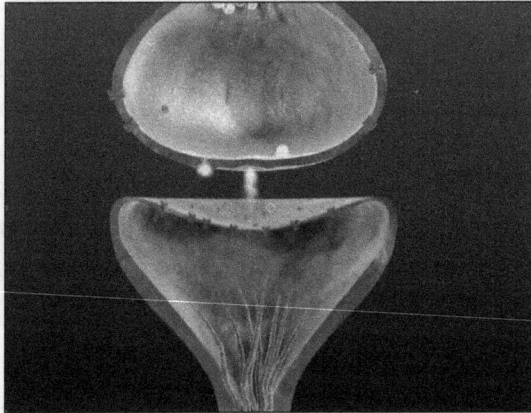

Figure 15. Neurotransmitters crossing the synaptic cleft between two nerve cells.
Image reprinted with permission from Purdu Pharma L.P. © 2002.

The main neurotransmitters in the intestines are norepinephrine, acetylcholine, dopamine, nitric oxide, and serotonin. There are even other chemicals in the gut that resemble psychoactive drugs like Valium® and Xanax®. Through many chemical interactions, *homeostasis* (balance) in the gut is maintained.

The neurotransmitter serotonin stimulates the peristaltic reflex. This reflex causes the wave-like motion in the gut muscles, pushing the waste products through the intestinal tract and out of the body. When serotonin is applied to the surface of the bowel, the peristaltic reflex is initiated. When serotonin is removed, the reflex is not as strong. In Hirschsprung's Disease, the absence of the nerves, serotonin, and other chemicals leads to a halt in peristalsis (Gershon, 1999).

CAUSES OF HIRSCHSPRUNG'S DISEASE

THERE ARE CURRENTLY three main theories as to the cause of Hirschsprung's Disease. The first and most popular theory is that there is a defect in the neural crest resulting in poor migration of nerve cells to the last part of the gut. The second theory holds that these nerve cells colonize the gut normally, but a toxic event caused the nerve cells to die in a certain region. The final theory suggests that the wall of the intestine is abnormal and unable to support these cells (Dranis, Staines, and Donat, 2005). I will examine the first and most popular theory in more detail.

The nervous system develops from cells that form a flat thickening on the back surface of the embryo. This thickening is called the neural plate and eventually develops into the nerve cells of the nervous system. As the embryo develops, the neural plate moves inward forming the neural groove and the neural folds. Eventually, the neural tube develops into the brain and spinal cord (see Figure 16).

Somewhere between the 5th and 12th week of pregnancy, the nerve cells form and migrate down the digestive tract of fetus. These nerve cells normally develop and implant themselves into the wall of the digestive tract from the mouth to the anus. In babies with Hirschsprung's Disease, the nerve cells stop migrating at a certain point in the intestines (the transition zone). Nothing the mother eats or takes as medication, has been shown to cause this problem. The disease is said to be congenital, meaning present at birth.

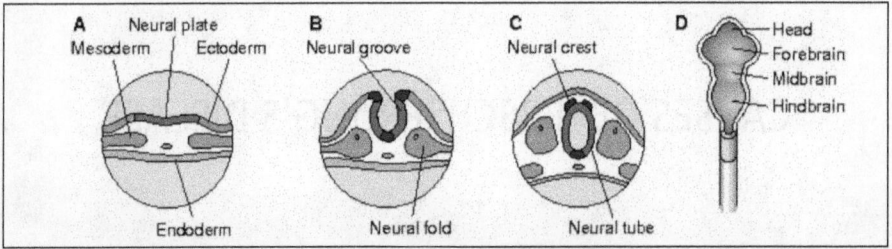

Figure 16. Neural crest stem cells develop underneath the ectoderm (skin).
Below is an actual photo of the neural tube that will eventually develop into a fetus.

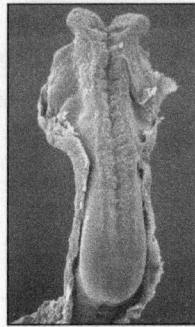

Image reprinted with permission from Deric Bownds, 2010.

Scientists at The University of Michigan (UM) Medical School in Ann Arbor have done extensive research on Hirschsprung's Disease. Based on new research, UM scientists now say the basic problem is that neural crest stem cells (NCSC), which give rise to nerves in the embryonic digestive system, never reach the lower part of the developing gut. Scientists have known for years that Hirschsprung's is a genetic disease and some gene *mutations* (changes in the genes of the cell) have been identified. Other scientists have found that these mutations can change the number of NCSCs, their survival rate, and their migration into the intestines.

Sean Morrison, PhD., directed research at the UM and found that the mutated genes causing HD occur in the neural crest cells themselves. As a result, the cells are not able to help form a normal digestive system. Embryonic stem cells can develop into any cell in the body. Neural crest stem cells only develop into the neurons and supporting cells of the peripheral nervous system. The NCSCs link the central nervous system and the peripheral nervous system together, allowing the brain to communicate with other parts of the body.

When all goes correctly, NCSCs migrate through the developing gut, and implant the digestive system with stem cells. These cells then help form a healthy digestive tract. In embryos with HD, some or all of these neural crest stem cells get stuck and cannot migrate to the last part of the digestive system (hind gut).

It is interesting to note that alterations in the development of the NCSCs result in an array of other human diseases such as: *Piebaldism* (two different eye colors), *albinism* (a lack of pigment in the skin), *melanoma* (mole cancer), *cleft lip and palate* (a malformation of the lip and palate), Hirschsprung's Disease, *neuroblastoma* (a malignant tumor occurring first in the abdomen around the adrenal gland), and others.

In their studies on mice and rats, scientists at the UM have also found that these neural crest stem cells remain in the gut of rats and mice throughout their adult lives. Morrison is hoping to transplant these cells from the upper to the lower gut of rats born with Hirschsprung's disease to see if it is possible to develop some functional nerves in the colon after birth. Dr. Morrison cautions that his research is based on findings in mice—not in humans yet. It could take years for scientists to know if this knowledge can be applied to humans.

DIAGNOSIS OF HIRSCHSPRUNG'S DISEASE

THE FIRST THING THE PEDIATRICIAN WILL DO when they suspect
Hirschsprung's Disease is an abdominal x-ray, specifically, a KUB (Kidneys, Ureters, and Bladder). The term KUB is a very old term and is just
another name for a plain abdominal film. The doctor may also order
an abdominal series, which includes x-rays of different angles of the
abdomen. The doctor will look for a low obstructive pattern, a lack of
gas in the rectum, and large dilated loops of intestine in the x-ray when
diagnosing Hirschsprung's Disease (see Figure 17). In most cases, the
next step in confirming HD would be a contrast enema.

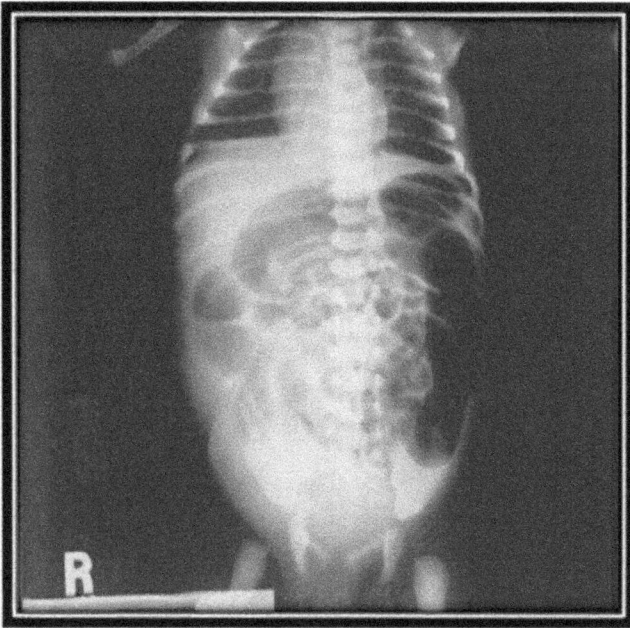

Figure 17. Abdominal x-ray (KUB) showing Hirschsprung's Disease.
Image reprinted with permission from Dr. Tom J. Curran. April 28, 2009.

Barium enema

A contrast or Barium enema is the second most common study ordered when Hirschsprung's Disease is suspected. A barium enema, or lower gastrointestinal (GI) examination, is an x-ray examination of the large intestine (colon and rectum). Barium is a non water-soluble agent that allows the doctor to see if there is narrowing or enlargement of the intestine. This metallic, chalky chemical is placed directly into the rectum. This liquid coats the inside of the intestines so they will show up on an x-ray. The contrast material is poured into a tube, which is inserted into the anus. The barium blocks the x-rays, allowing the barium-filled colon to show up clearly on the x-ray picture (WebMD, 2009).

In cases with HD, there will usually be *stricture* (narrowing), obstruction (blockage), and a dilated intestine above the obstruction. An irregular "saw tooth" appearance of the rectum (see Figure 18), as well as a cone-shaped narrowing from the megacolon to the aganglionic rectum can also be a valuable signs of Hirschsprung's Disease in a barium x-ray (Nixon, 1985).

Gastrografin

In some children with HD, it is difficult to rid the colon of the barium. In these cases, a substance called gastrografin is used. Gastrografin is an x-ray dye that can be swallowed or put through an NG tube into the stomach.

The iodine in the gastrografin allows the doctor to see what section or sections of the colon may be affected by Hirschsprung's Disease. Gastrografin is water-soluble and is not absorbed into the bloodstream but draws water from the walls of the intestine, causing diarrhea. Gastrografin is now more commonly used in children with Hirschsprung's Disease because it can be passed through the intestinal tract more easily and has very few side effects (Drugs.com, 2006).

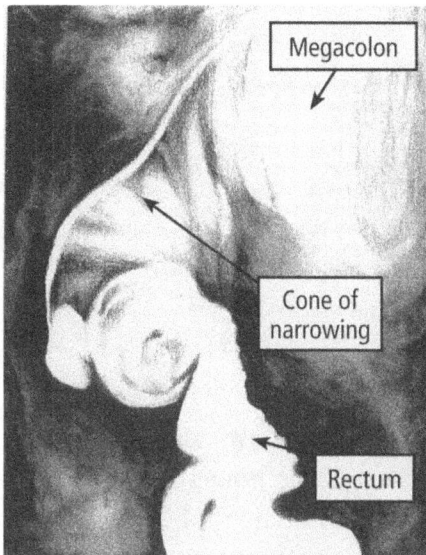

Figure 18. Barium Enema cone of narrowing.
Illustration by Mackenzie Edlund, 2011.

Suction biopsy and full-thickness biopsy

The surgeon will perform a suction biopsy in a newborn with suspected HD. Suction rectal biopsies work best in small infants, generally up to about one year of age. This is a painless procedure for the baby. During the biopsy, the doctor removes a tiny piece of the intestine using a special device. It does not require anesthesia. The piece of intestine is then observed under a microscope to see if the nerve cells are missing in the tissue. If the nerve cells are missing, then Hirschsprung's Disease is the problem (see Figures 19 and 20).

In older children, suction rectal biopsies are not as reliable, so a full-thickness biopsy, where more of the colon tissue is collected, may be required. General anesthesia is used during a full-thickness biopsy. Full-thickness biopsies are extremely accurate in the diagnosis of Hirschsprung's Disease.

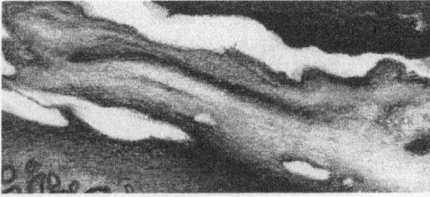

Figure 19. Biopsy showing HD.	Figure 20. Biopsy showing no HD.
No nerve cells are present	Nerve cells are present.

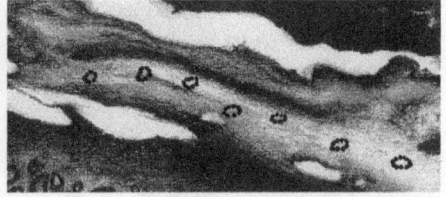

Illustrations by Mackenzie Edlund, 2011.

Diagnosing long-segment HD and total colonic HD

Diagnosis for long-segment HD can also be difficult. X-rays may show multiple enlarged loops of the bowel throughout the abdomen and a question mark-shaped colon. The problem with the x-rays is that they can only be used to diagnose this form of HD in 20% to 30% of patients afflicted with it. Most often, the diagnosis of LSHD is made during the operation for the colostomy. The surgeons will also look for ganglion cells in the appendix. If they are absent, then long-segment HD can be confirmed.

There are three critical phases for patients with total colonic aganglionosis/HD (TCA). The first phase is from the time of birth until correct diagnosis. Children with TCA have a large variety of symptoms leading to a delayed diagnosis. The mortality rates among these children are higher because they usually have more surgeries and have more episodes of *enterocolitis* (infection in the colon).

Other complications include: failure to grow, *stomal* (opening for the colostomy bag) dysfunctions, electrolyte imbalance, dehydration, and organ failure from the special parenteral feedings these children have. The parenteral feeding (total parenteral nutrition or TPN) is done by way of a special IV, which can become infected over time. This infection can get into the bloodstream *(sepsis)*, which can be deadly.

TYPES OF HIRSCHSPRUNG'S DISEASE

THE FIVE MAIN TYPES OF HIRSCHSPRUNG'S DISEASE are ultra-short segment HD, short-segment HD, long-segment HD, total colonic HD, near total intestinal, and total intestinal HD. Intestinal neuronal dysplasia (IND) is a disorder that is similar to ultra-short HD.

Ultra-short segment HD

Ultra-short segment HD occurs when there is only about a 2 to 4 cm segment of the rectum near the anus that shows no nerve cells (see Figure 21). This can be confusing for doctors and clinicians because it is rare, and many times the rectal biopsy may show ganglion cells. Many children with this type of HD have chronic constipation and fecal soiling. There can be other causes of these problems, making it difficult to confirm an HD diagnosis.

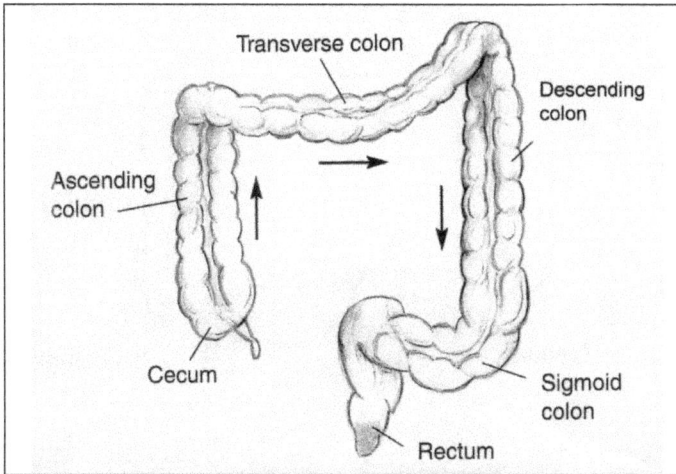

Figure 21. Ultra-short segment Hirschsprung's Disease shown in shaded area.

Image reprinted with permission from The National Institute of Diabetes and Digestive and Kidney Diseases, National Institute of Health, 2010.

Generally, a contrast enema (x-ray with a barium enema/gastro-grafin) is used to show the transition zone in Hirschsprung's Disease; however, it may not be an accurate test for ultra-short HD. Many children with ultra-short HD may be overlooked because it is not routine in many medical centers to perform an anorectal manometry. For children with ultra-short segment HD, problems with constipation and soiling can be life-long.

Short-segment HD

Short-segment Hirschsprung's Disease (SSHD) is the most common form of HD. Ultra-short and short-segment HD occur in about 80% of the cases according to Edery, Pelet, Mulligan, Abel, Attie, Dow Bonneau, David, Flintoff, and Jan (1994). It is limited to the rectum and the sigmoid colon or recto-sigmoid area (see Figure 22). In other words, if the diseased section is only part of the large intestine, it is short-segment HD. This form of Hirschsprung's Disease is multi-factorial, meaning it takes the interaction of many genes to cause it.

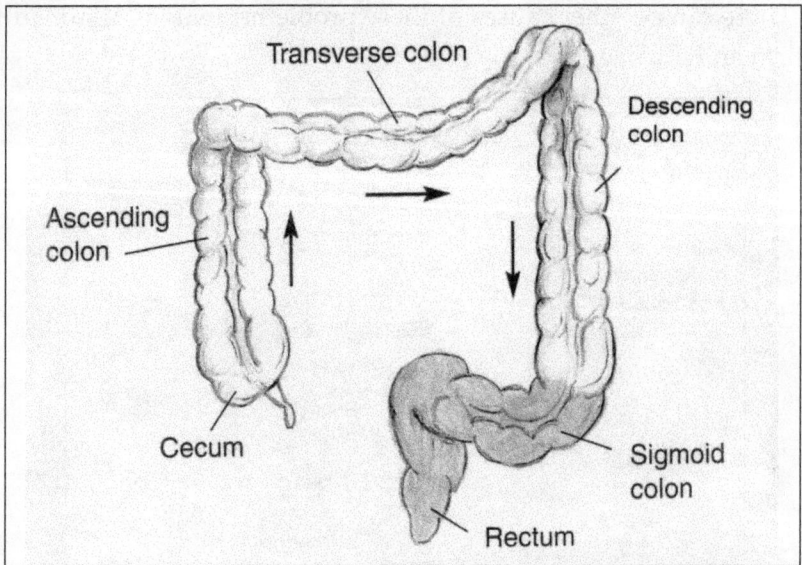

Figure 22. Short-segment Hirschsprung's Disease shown in shaded area.
Image reprinted with permission from The National Institute of Diabetes and Digestive and Kidney Diseases, National Institute of Health, 2010.

Long-segment HD

If the diseased portion of the bowel involves more than half of the colon (past the splenic flexure), Long-segment Hirschsprung's Disease is diagnosed (LSHD) (see Figure 23).

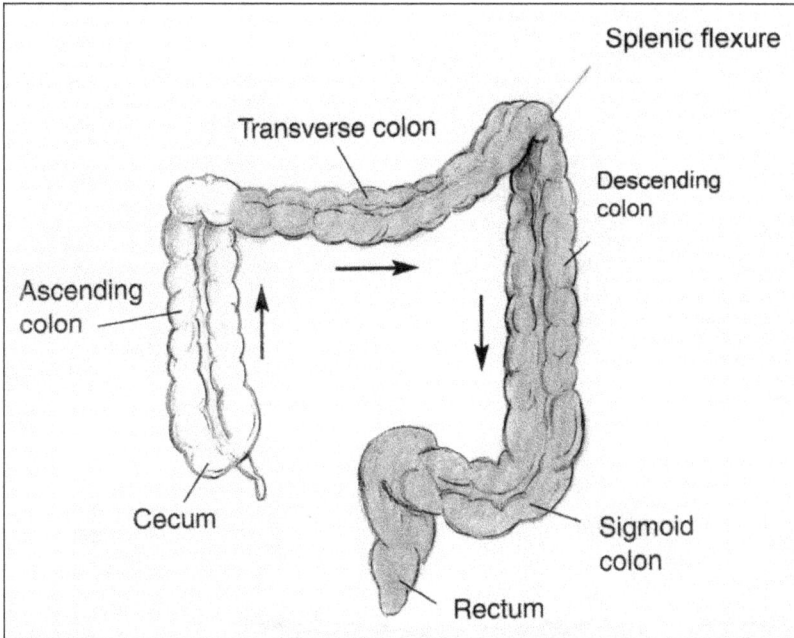

Figure 23. Long-segment Hirschsprung's Disease shown in shaded area.

Image reprinted with permission from The National Institute of Diabetes and Digestive and Kidney Diseases, National Institute of Health, 2010.

Total Colonic Aganglionosis (TCA) or
Total Colonic Hirschsprung's Disease (TCHD)

Total colonic aganglionosis (TCA) occurs in 5% of children with Hirschsprung's Disease (Teitelbaum, Coran, Wetizman, 1998). This means that all of the large intestine is without the nerve cells, which initiate peristalsis (see Figure 24).

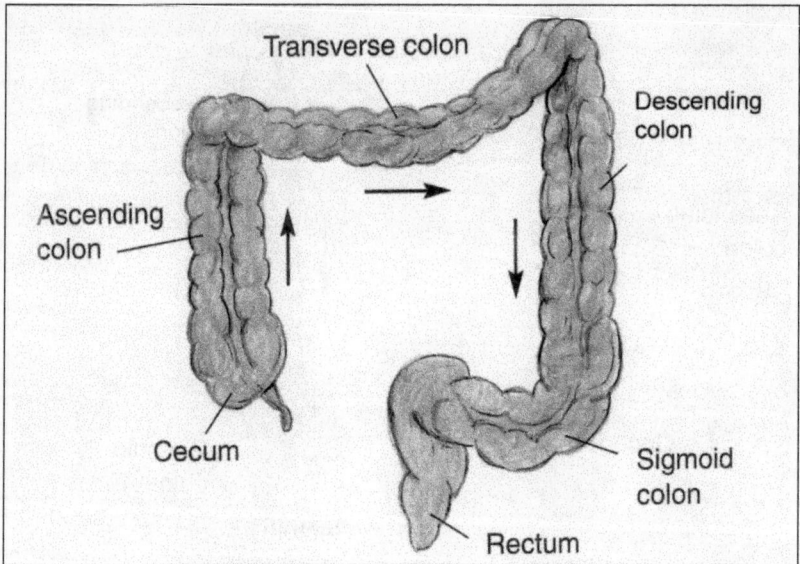

Figure 24. Total colonic Hirschsprung's Disease shown in shaded area.

Image reprinted with permission from The National Institute of Diabetes and Digestive and Kidney Diseases, National Institute of Health, 2010.

Near total intestinal Hirschsprung's Disease (NTIHD) or near total intestinal aganglionosis (NTIA).

Near total HD occurs when aganglionosis involves at least 40 cm of the jejunum (the next 2.5m of small intestine past the duodenum) (Ziegler & Royal, 1993). Between the years 1974 and 1999 patients with NTIA were a part of a study to determine their long-term outcomes. Seven full-term babies were identified. All seven were diagnosed within the first five days of life.

The conclusion of the study was that aganglionosis involving most of the bowel has a high *morbidity* (illness as a result of the disease) and *mortality* rate (death from disease). However, since 1990, a more aggressive surgical approach (extended jejunal myotomy or myectomy) has resulted in improved survival rates for these children (Saxton, Ein, Heohner, & Kim, 2000).

Total intestinal Hirschsprung's Disease (TIHD) or Total intestinal Aganglionosis (TIA)

Otherwise known as total aganglionosis, total intestinal Hirschsprung's Disease occurs when the nerve cells are lacking from the stomach to the rectum. Total aganglionosis is rare and occurs in less than 5-10% of all reported cases of Hirschsprung's Disease (Kleinhaus & Boley, 1979) and (Ikeda & Goto, 1984).

Intestinal transplantation

Across the globe, 65 centers have performed 1,292 small bowel transplants with a five-year survival rate of 50% or better. Thirteen years is the longest any patients have survived following a small bowel transplant (Longworth &Young, 2006). The most frequent source for small bowel donors is from cadavers, but some living donors have also been used (Testa, et al. 1998).

The digestive tract is amazing in that only the small bowel is essential for survival. The parts of the *small bowel* (duodenum, jejunum, and ileum) each have different functions. Digestion mainly occurs in the *duodenum* (the first 25 cm of the small intestine). *Enzymes* (proteins that speed up chemical reactions in the body) are released into the duodenum from the pancreas and the liver to digest proteins, fats, and carbohydrates. After the duodenum has broken down most of the *chyme* (digesting food), the *jejunum* (the following 2.5 m) allows these nutrients to be absorbed into the blood stream. Because the pores in the ileum (the remaining 3.5 m of small intestine) are slightly larger than those in the jejunum, vitamins, electrolytes, and water can soak through the walls and into the blood stream. The blood stream then carries the nutrients to various parts of the body for different uses.

Patients can survive losing many parts of the digestive system, however loss of the small intestines requires external feedings by way of total parenteral nutrition (TPN). Interestingly, it has been observed that after several months, many patients who require TPN can be supported either partially or totally with oral feedings. This suggests that whatever small bowel remains can actually improve in function over time (Weale & Edwards, 2005).

OPERATIONS FOR HIRSCHSPRUNG'S DISEASE

BEFORE SURGERY FOR HD, the patient's intestines are decompressed; meaning all of the material in the intestines is washed out along with the gas. An NG tube may be put through the nostril and down into the stomach. A fluid called GoLYTELY® is then run through it. This is a laxative that gets rid of everything in the intestines so that the surgeon can see what he or she is doing during the operation. The parent may have to perform irrigations to help rid the intestines of feces because babies with HD cannot get their stool out on their own.

Once the intestines have been successfully decompressed, the pull-through or colostomy operation can be performed. In some cases, the surgeon will have the parents do home rectal irrigations for weeks or months prior to the surgery. This approach is preferable because it allows the baby to increase in size before surgery. In other cases, it is necessary for the baby to have surgery right away (IPEG, 2005).

Staged surgical approach

Depending on the severity of the Hirschsprung's Disease, either a primary pull-through or a two-stage operation will be performed. If a staged approach is planned, the surgeon will first remove the diseased part of the intestine. Then, the doctor cuts a small hold in the baby's abdomen. This hole is called a *stoma*.

The doctor then connects the top part of the intestine to the stoma. The stool leaves the body through the stoma while the bottom part of the intestine heals. It is at this point where the colostomy bag will be attached to the patient. The bag will then need to be emptied several times daily.

Ileostomy/colostomy

The five types of ostomies are; an ileostomy, an ascending colostomy, a transverse colostomy, a descending colostomy, and a sigmoid colostomy (see Figure 25). If the entire large intestine is removed, the surgery is called an *ileostomy*. It is called this because the *ileum* (last part of the small intestine before the large intestine) becomes the stoma. If the doctor leaves part of the large intestine and connects that to the stoma, the surgery is called a *colostomy* (NIDDK, 2003). If the ascending or descending section of the colon is attached to the stoma, it is called an *ascending/descending* colostomy. When the surgeon connects the *transverse colon* (part of colon which connects the ascending colon to the descending colon) to the stoma, the procedure is a *transverse colostomy*. Likewise, when the *sigmoid colon* (s-shaped area of colon above rectum) is connected to the stoma, the procedure is called a *sigmoid colostomy*. The surgeon will decide which type of ostomy is best for the patient. If possible, after a few months, the patient will have a second surgery to pull down and reattach the healthy bowel and the stoma will be closed.

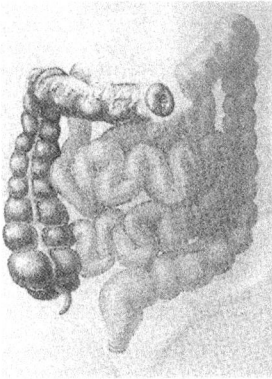 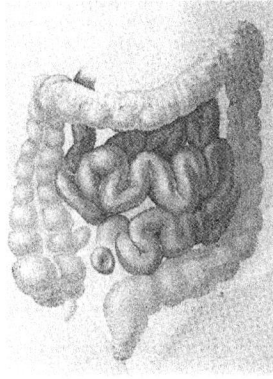 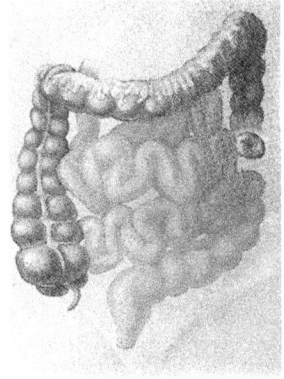

| Transverse colostomy | Ileostomy | Ileostomy |

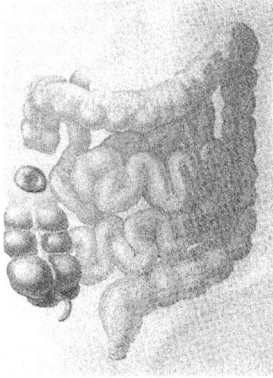 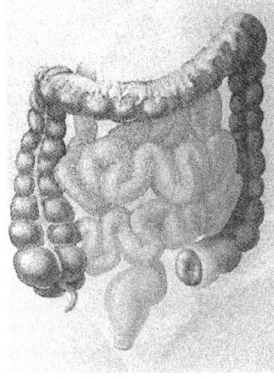

Ascending colostomy   Sigmoid Colostomy

Figure 25. Types of ostomies.

Images reprinted with permission from the International Foundation for Functional Gastrointestinal Disorders (IFFG). © 2007. www.aboutkidsgi.org

Laparoscopic surgery

Laparoscopic surgery is a minimally invasive surgery in which the surgeon uses a scope and monitor to locate and remove the diseased bowel. Three or more incisions are made in the abdomen to allow the surgeon to place the scope inside of the abdomen. With this procedure, there is rapid recovery and less external and internal scarring (IPEG, 2005).

Primary pull-through

Years ago, surgery for Hirschsprung's Disease was always done in two stages. Now, surgeons agree that when possible, it is most beneficial to perform the operation in one stage in the neonate period (just after birth or shortly after). This operation is called a *primary pull-through* (see Figure 26), and most types can be done *open* (with external incision), *laparoscopically*, or *transanally* (through the anus).

Children without evidence of severe *enterocolitis* (infection in the colon) are good candidates for this procedure. Studies have shown a decrease in illness and death when surgery is performed earlier in Hirschsprung's patients (Wilcox, Bruce, Bowen, and Bianchi, 1997). Currently, there are three commonly used procedures to treat Hirschsprung's Disease. They are the Swenson, Soave, and Duhamel methods.

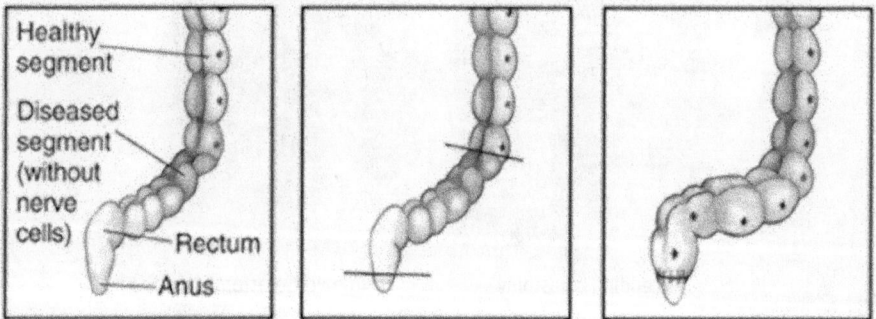

Figure 26. Diseased section is removed during a Primary Pull-Through Operation. The rectum is largely removed and only a small portion above the anus remains. The healthy section is then attached to the remaining rectum (Bliss, 2005).

The Swenson and Bill procedure

In 1948, Orvar Swenson and Alexander Bill developed the first operation to treat Hirschsprung's Disease. Swenson performed a sigmoid colostomy on a five-year-old child. One year later, he closed the colostomy and the child's symptoms returned. It was then that Swenson decided to remove the aganglionic section of the colon and reattach the remaining healthy colon to the rectum. Once again, the symptoms cleared and the child survived.

In this operation, the surgeon will keep the dissection next to the rectal wall to avoid injury to the pelvic nerves responsible for bladder control and sexual function (American Pediatric Surgical Association (APSA), 2003). Orvar Swenson was a pioneer in surgery for Hirschsprung's Disease and invested many years researching this disorder (see Figure 27).

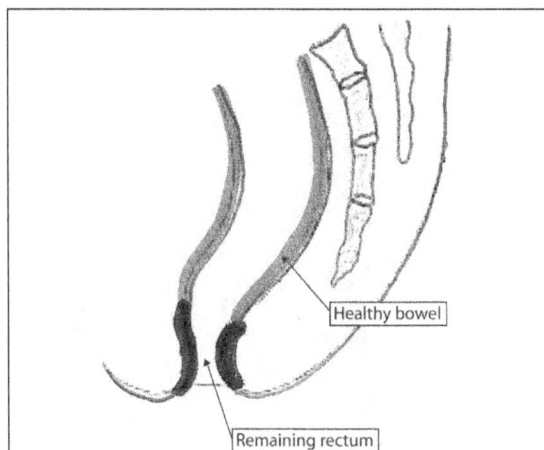

Figure 27. The Swenson Procedure.
Bold black lines indicate the part of the rectum that remains, and the shaded area indicates the healthy bowel that has been pulled down and reattached.

Illustration by Nicole Murphy, 2010

The Duhamel procedure

Devised by French doctor Bernard Duhamel in 1956, this procedure is done more frequently in Europe and is essentially the same as the Swenson and Soave (ASPA, 2003). The main difference between the other two methods and the Duhamel is that the normal bowel is brought down behind the rectum and the end of this bowel is sewn to the side of the rectum near the anus (see Figure 28).

Finally, the pulled-through bowel is stapled with a special surgical staple to the rectum. Now, the patient has a new rectum with the front half made-up of the aganglionic rectum and the back half made-up of the new pulled-through healthy colon. The front of the bowel will have no ganglion cells, but the back will be healthy (Sawin, 2005).

The benefit of this surgery is that it is minimally invasive in the pelvic area, which contains many important nerves. The main drawbacks to this surgery are stool retention and a high incontinence rate. This is because of the long rectal section that is left during the operation. Another advantage of this operation, is that it is easier to perform and can be done when other procedures have failed.

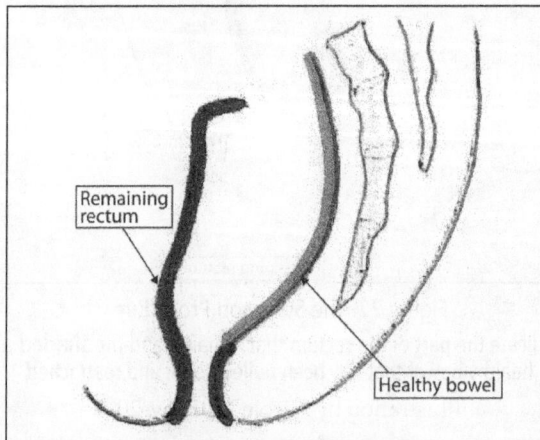

Figure 28. The Duhamel procedure.
The bold black lines indicate the part of the rectum that remains, and the shaded area indicates the healthy bowel that has been pulled down and reattached.
Illustration by Nicole Murphy, 2010

The Soave procedure

The Soave procedure was introduced in 1960 (see Figure 29). During this procedure, the *mucosa* (lining) of the rectum is removed as well as the diseased section of the colon. This operation is also called an endorectal pull-through.

The healthy portion of the colon is then brought down through the rectal cuff, and sewn to the inside of the cuff just above the anal sphincters. Pediatric Surgeon, Dr. Tom Curran, likens it to two pipes being connected. Theoretically, leaving behind aganglionic muscle surrounding the normal bowel might lead to a higher incidence of constipation. This, however, has not been the case (Sawin, 2005).

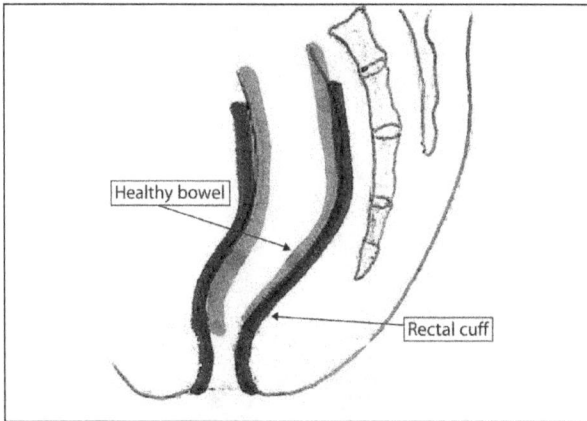

Figure 29. The Soave procedure.
The bold black lines indicate the part of the rectum that remains and the shaded area indicates the healthy bowel that has been pulled down and reattached to the rectal cuff.
Illustration by Nicole Murphy, 2010

Dr. Sawin, an expert in pull-through surgery, notes, "Although there are about five different pull-through procedures, they are all more or less equally effective in treating the disorder" (Sawin, 2005). He also states, "85% of patients that have the pull-through surgery live normal lives afterwards. The other 15% have to take a laxative for the rest of their lives." In cases of total HD, there are no ganglion cells at all in the colon and a Martin pull-through operation is conducted (Sawin, 2005). This operation requires a colostomy no matter how early the HD is diagnosed.

WHAT TO EXPECT AFTER THE OPERATION

ALL SURGERY CARRIES A SMALL RISK of bleeding during or after the operation. There is a small chance that the bowel could leak into the abdominal cavity causing an infection called peritonitis. If this should occur, the child would need a stoma, which would deter infection. In more severe cases of HD, it is necessary that the child be placed on long-term TPN (See appendix for TPN line care).

There is also a chance that the blood supply to the newly pulled-through colon is insufficient, or that the colon was pulled-through too tightly. This results in a stricture or scarring of the *anastomosis* (point at which the colon is reconnected to the rectum), which then causes the colon to stop functioning properly. It will be necessary to have the operation redone in the cases discussed above. Other surgical risks include the need for a blood transfusion, incontinence, constipation, impotence, and *retrograde ejaculation* (occurs when the semen to be ejaculated, which would normally exit through the urethra, is redirected towards the urinary bladder).

Every time a person goes under anesthesia, there is a small risk of complications. Luckily, pediatric anesthesiologists are very experienced doctors who are highly trained to deal with any emergencies. A pull-through operation can last anywhere from 2-8 hours; about halfway through the operation, the surgical nurse will brief the parents on how the surgery is going.

What to expect after surgery

After surgery, the child is brought back into either the NICU or the Pediatric Unit, depending on his/her age. The child may be on a respirator and will be monitored closely by the nurses in the unit. After awhile, the child will be taken off of the respirator and kept comfortable with pain medications. It is important to have a notebook handy to write down which pain medications worked well for the child and which ones did not. In some cases, children with HD require more than one operation, so this written information could come in handy at a later date.

Doctor visits after surgery

During these examinations, the surgeon will check the anastomosis by doing a rectal exam, and will ask the parents questions about stooling frequency and consistency. The surgeon will insert a gloved finger into the anus to be sure that everything has healed properly. Usually, this causes the baby to have a bowel movement and can cause a little bleeding.

If necessary, the surgeon will explain how to do the dilatations and irrigations. *(Sometimes, the surgeon will refer to the dilatations as dilations just because it is easier to say).* During a dilatation, a *dilator* (metal or plastic rod) is inserted into the anus. This keeps the anastomosis from closing. The diameter of the dilator is increased until the opening is sufficient for bowel movements to occur easily (see Figure 30). For guidelines on how to perform a dilatation and irrigation, please refer to the appendix.

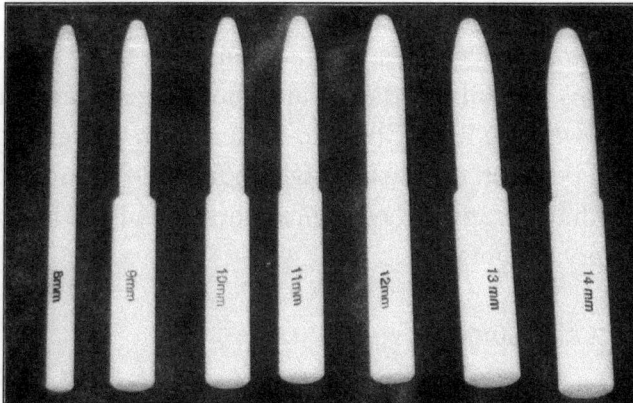

Figure 30. Dilators shown in ascending size.
Image reprinted with permission from Hirschsprungshelp@yahoo.com , 2010.

In some cases, it will be necessary to do rectal irrigations to keep the colon clean. A *decompression tube* (long rubber tube used to rinse out the colon) is inserted into the colon after it has been lubricated with a special jell, usually KY Jelly (see Figure 31). As the baby lies on a sterile pad, saline solution is squirted into the tube via a large syringe. The irrigations keep harmful bacteria from building up in the colon and also allow gas to be released. Every surgeon has different techniques, so it is important to check with the doctor to be sure the irrigations are being done properly.

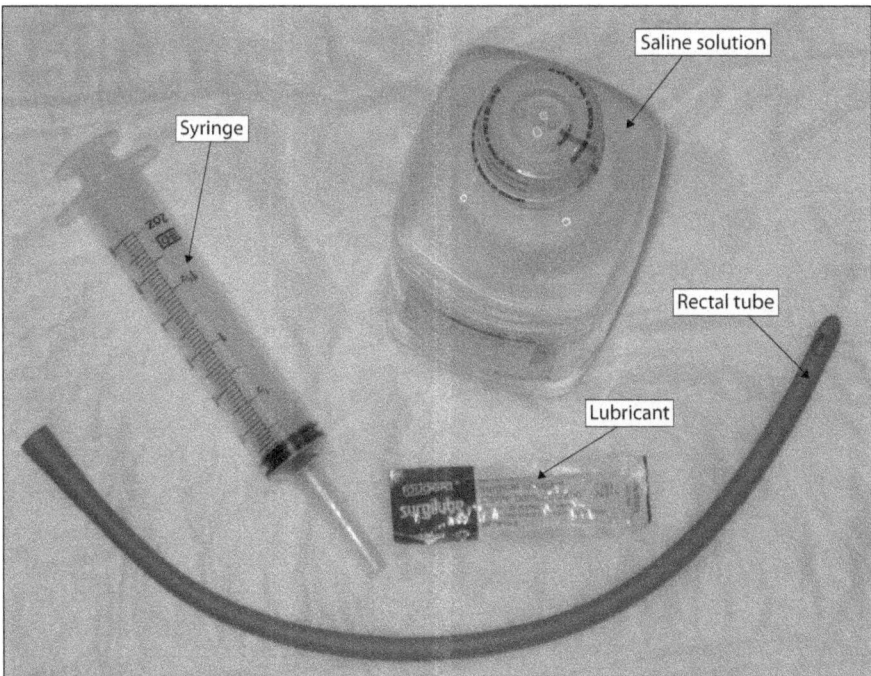

Figure 31. Rectal tube, sterile pad, saline solution, lubricant, and syringe.
Image reprinted with permission from Hirschsprungshelp@yahoo.com, 2010.

DILATATION & IRRIGATION GUIDELINES

IT TAKES TWO ADULTS to do a dilatation and irrigation, one to hold the baby, and one to perform the procedure (see Figure 32). Also, if the parent can prepare the area before bringing the baby in, it will lessen the time the baby has to be upset.

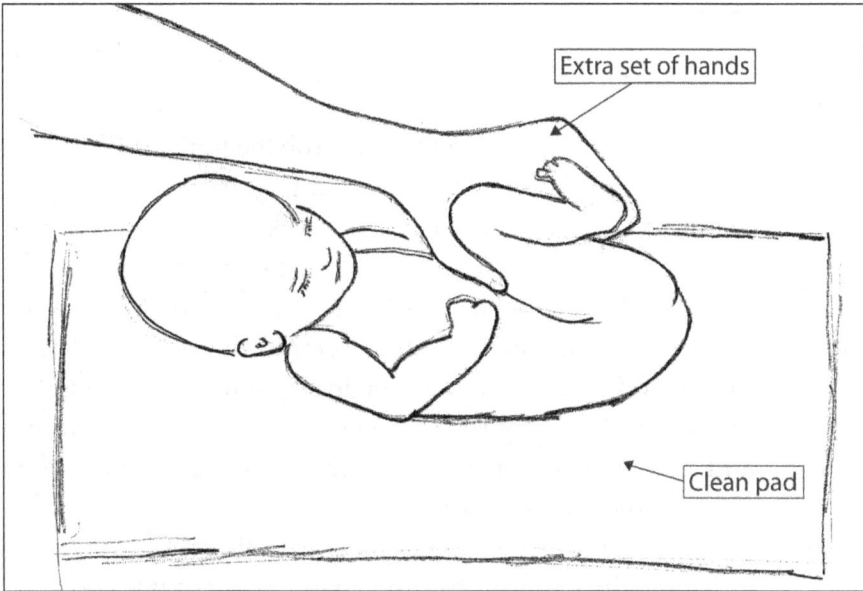

Figure 32. How to hold a baby's legs during an irrigation and dilatation.
Illustration by Margie Baxter. © 2006.

Dilatation

1. Wash the dilatation rod and irrigation tube with warm soapy water and then dry.
2. Squirt some lubricating jelly onto the disposable bed pad.
3. Fill the syringe with saline to the designated line

4. Place the baby onto the pad and bring his/her knees up toward the chest.
5. Hold firmly and talk reassuringly to your baby. This helps to distract him/her during the dilatation.
6. Put the dilator into the lubricating jelly and liberally cover the end of it.
7. Gently insert the lubricated dilator into the anus - about 2-3 inches in. Then retract the dilator (*not all of the way out of the anus*) and then insert it again. Finally, remove the dilator totally. Ask the surgeon to explain this in detail.
8. The baby should have a bowel movement at this point and may also release some gas.

Irrigation

1. While continuing to hold the baby, roll the tubing end into the lubricating jelly and coat well (about 2-3 inches of the tip).
2. Gently insert the tubing until you feel it stop. Draw a permanent line onto the tubing so as not to puncture the colon.
3. Once you feel the tube stop inject the saline solution into the other end of the rubber tubing. Remove the syringe from the tubing and then move the tube in and out slightly to get rid of the gas. Then, squirt the rest of the saline into the tubing and move it again in and out slightly. The stool should come out the other end of the tube.
4. Keeping the tube in the colon, repeat this procedure one or two more times. The tube can slip out easily so it is necessary to have someone hold the tube in the colon until the irrigation is finished.
5. Once the fluid coming out of the rectum is clear, the parent can be sure that the colon is clean. About the same amount of saline should come out as went in.
6. After the baby has been cleaned, pick him/her up and comfort them. This can be a very traumatic experience for the baby.

How long do the irrigations & dilatations have to be done?

Once the baby starts pooping on his/her own, the irrigations can usually be stopped. Be sure to talk with the surgeon about this. If the baby starts to have smelly green stools, begin the irrigations again—this can signal the beginning of enterocolitis. If the feces is not freely flowing but chunky as it comes out, this could indicate constipation.

If constipation is the problem, a laxative called MiraLax® will bring more water into the colon and will soften the stool so that the child can pass it more easily. Generally, once a laxative is introduced, the child can be done with the irrigations. It is very important to have the decompression tube available during the stomach flu—or a bout of enterocolitis. If the child needs to be hospitalized, bring all of the supplies along. Use an old diaper bag and just have it handy in case it is necessary to rush out the door to the hospital. Also, if the baby needs an upper GI at any time, bring the tube along as children with HD can have a hard time passing the Gastrografin or barium.

DIAPER RASH AFTER A PULL-THROUGH OPERATION

AFTER A PULL-THROUGH OPERATION, the loose and acidic stools can cause a severe diaper rash. This is especially true in babies who have no colon (TCA), to absorb water, leaving the ileum to learn this function. When moisture from the urine and stool sits on the sensitive skin, it breaks down. Fungus (yeast) and bacteria from the stool and intestines can thrive in this moist environment. In children with HD, it is important to prevent a bad diaper rash because they will begin to associate pain upon defecation. This can then cause children with HD to have other issues, such as stool holding, which will lead to constipation.

Once the baby has been brought home from the hospital, it is crucial to keep the diaper rash under control. ILEX© cream (see Figure 33) is the most widely used barrier ointment after a pull-through operation. Proshield© Plus skin protectant can be used over the ILEX© to provide extra protection from acidic stools.

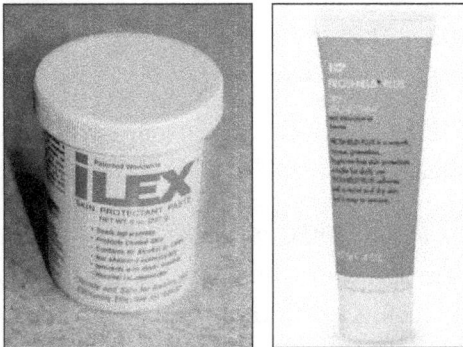

Figure 33. ILEX© skin protectant and Proshield© Plus

Image reprinted with permission from www.woundcareshop.com. © 2010

Types of diaper rashes

- *Yeast rash*

When yeast from the intestines invades the damaged skin it causes a red bumpy rash (see Figure 34). This rash covers the genitalia with satellite lesions (scattered spots) around the diaper area. *Candidal organisms* (fungus) cause a yeast rash. This usually occurs when the environment is warm and moist, like in diaper areas and skin folds. Antibiotics can kill the naturally occurring bacteria on the skin that keep the yeast in check, allowing the yeast to multiply around the diaper area. Yeast rashes may cause itching or pain and are very common in children with HD after a pull-through operation (AskDrSears.com, 2006).

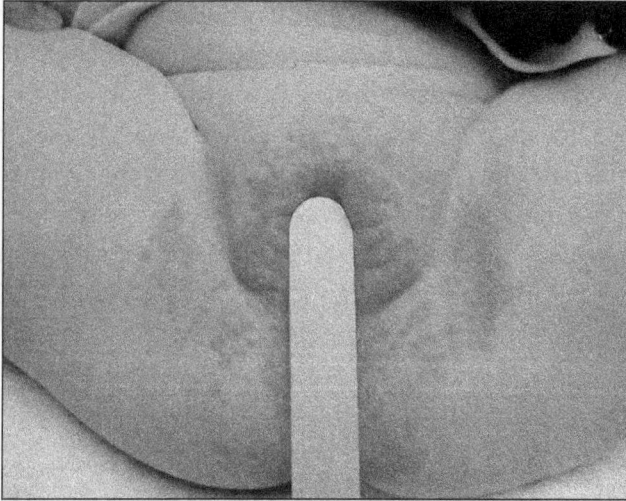

Figure 34. Bumpy patches associated with a yeast diaper rash.
Image reprinted with permission from AskDrSears.com, © 2006.

Treatment for a yeast rash: Clotrimazole (an over-the-counter medication), *Nystatin* (prescription medication), and a 1% hydrocortisone cream can also be applied to reduce inflammation. Acidophilus is a natural bacterial powder that fights off yeast. It can be purchased at most health food stores.

- *Contact diaper rash*

A common rash that appears flat and red (see Figure 35). In severe cases, the skin can peel or blister and slough off.

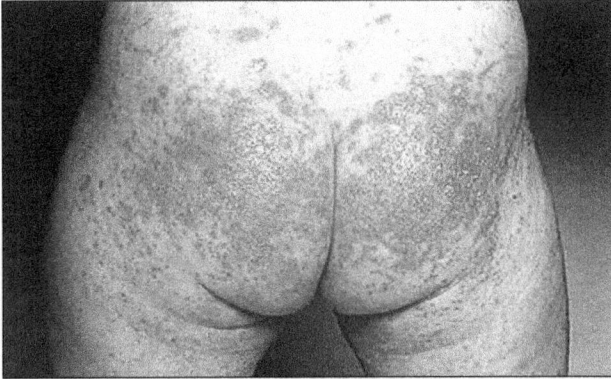

Figure 35. Prolonged exposure to urine or stool can cause a contact diaper rash.
Image reprinted with permission from the Mayo Foundation for Medical Education and Research, © 2007.

Treatment for a contact diaper rash: A barrier ointment like Aquaphor® or Zinc oxide will keep urine and feces away from the skin so that it can begin to heal. In more severe cases, ILEX© cream is very effective.

- *Allergy ring*

Some foods can irritate the skin on the bottom, especially acidic foods like tomato-based sauces and citrus fruits.

Treatment for allergy ring: Stop using suspected foods. Moms who are breastfeeding may need to eliminate certain foods from their diet.

HIRSCHSPRUNG ASSOCIATED ENTEROCOLITIS (HAEC)

THE SYMPTOMS OF ENTEROCOLITIS are explosive diarrhea, swollen abdomen, vomiting, bleeding from the rectum, sluggishness, complete lack of bowel movements, and fever. Enterocolitis is defined as an inflammation of the lining of the colon or small intestine. As the disease gets worse, the lining of the intestine/colon erodes and the inside of the intestine becomes filled with pus. If a child exhibits any or all of these symptoms, the child should be taken to the doctor immediately. This infection can cause *perforation* (puncture) of the colon and death (see Figure 36).

Grade	Clinical symptoms
I	Mild explosive diarrhea, mild or moderate abdominal distension and no systemic manifestations (other symptoms in the body such as a fever).
II	Moderate explosive diarrhea, moderate to severe abdominal distention, and mild systemic manifestations.
III	Severe explosive diarrhea, marked abdominal distention, and shock or impending shock.

Figure 36. Clinical grading system showing varying degrees of HAEC by E.A. Elhalaby.
Table adapted with permission from Badner, et al.
The American Journal of Human Genetics 46: 569-580 (1990).

Factors that contribute to enterocolitis include poor movement of the intestinal contents, a bacterial invasion of the wall of the intestine, a decrease in the immune system in the intestines, and abnormal mucous secretions from the intestine. Enterocolitis may happen before or after a pull-through operation. This form of enterocolitis is known as Hirschsprung's associated enterocolitis (HAEC) and can occur with an excessively tight pull-through, or spasms of the anal sphincter.

Bill and Chapman were the first to describe the clinical aspects of HAEC (Bill & Chapman, 1962). They felt that the cause of the disorder was a partial mechanical obstruction. If repeated bouts of enterocolitis occur after the pull-through operation, then the surgeon should suspect the cause to be a mechanical problem (Teitelbaum, Qualman, and Caniano, 1988).

The two times an infant is at highest risk for HAEC is either before the Hirschsprung's diagnosis or following the pull-through operation (Surana, Qinn, and Puri, 1994). Parents should also be aware that there are varying degrees of enterocolitis and the child does not have to have all of the symptoms to need treatment. Many cases of diarrhea or abdominal distention may be mistakenly diagnosed as *gastroenteritis* (stomach flu), but most of these are cases of mild HAEC (Elhalaby, Teitelbaum, Coran, and Heidelberger, 1995). According to Dr. David Bliss at Emanuel Children's Hospital in Portland, Oregon, parents can usually stop worrying about HAEC when the child reaches about three years of age.

Clostridium difficile (C diff) is a bacterium that is commonly found in the intestinal tract. Normally, this bacterium is not harmful but can sometimes grow out of control and cause severe illness. It is believed that some Hirschsprung associated enterocolitis is caused by C diff. If HAEC is suspected, the doctor will obtain fecal samples from the affected patient. Clostridium difficile releases toxins into the stool, which can be detected by the tests run on the feces. If these toxins are present, then the doctor can diagnose HAEC. Immediately, antibiotics will be given to stop the course of the illness. In a study conducted by Thomas, Fernie, Bayston, Spitz, and Nixon (1986), it was found that children with HAEC had significantly greater C diff toxins in their stool as compared to the control group of children with no HAEC.

Infants with Down syndrome (Trisomy 21), have an increased risk of developing HAEC (Teitelbaum, Caniano, and Qualman, 1990).

In one study on HAEC, almost 45% of infants with Down syndrome and HD developed HAEC (Caniano, et al. 1988). Most likely, there is an increased immune deficiency in Downs babies (Levin, 1987). Other anomalies can also place the infant at risk for the development of enterocolitis. Caneiro, Brereton, Drake, Kiely, Spitz, and Turnock (1992) found that 53% of infants with other Hirschsprung associated anomalies, including Down syndrome, developed HAEC as compared to only 26% with HD alone.

Reoccurring HAEC is a problem for many children with HD after a pull-through operation. Patients who have an altered immune response like those with Down syndrome are especially susceptible to chronic HAEC. Although the frequency of enterocolitis tends to decrease over time, a small proportion of patients continue to have ongoing symptoms (Fortuna, Weber, and Tracey, 1996). Currently, the reason why this occurs is poorly understood.

In one study conducted by researchers at the Children's Hospital, University of Helsinki, Finland, it was found that sodium cromoglycate (SCG) significantly reduced symptoms of enterocolitis in some patients. Significant clinical improvement was noted in six of the eight patients being treated with SCG (Rintala, & Lindahl, 2001). SCG is also used to treat allergies and irritable bowel syndrome (IBS). Sodium cromoglycate is also called cromalyn or Gastrocrom®.

Treatment for HAEC consists of aggressive rectal irrigations or washouts using a large rectal tube to decompress the colon every four to six hours. Antibiotics like Flagyl® are given through an IV if enterocolitis is suspected. Blood and fecal tests are also done to rule out certain bacteria and viruses like C-diffcil and rotavirus. Abdominal x-rays can be helpful sometimes, but a contrast enema is more accurate. The only problem with doing a contrast enema during a bout of enterocolitis is that there is an increased risk for perforation of the colon.

PROBLEMS WITH DEFECATION AFTER SURGERY FOR HIRSCHSPRUNG'S DISEASE

MORE THAN 1,000 NEW CASES OF HD are diagnosed in the U.S. every year. After surgery for HD, many children suffer from incontinence, constipation, and abdominal pain. According to Cato-Smith, Coffey, Nolat, and Hutson, (1995) more than 50% experience incontinence (inability to control bowel movements) and 20% endure constipation (Di Lorenzo, et al. 2000). According to Dr. Paul Hyman of the University of Kansas Medical Center, the children are not lazy or uncooperative, but have real physiological reasons for their symptoms.

A child may suffer from constipation following a pull-through operation. Some of the reasons for this include a pull-through done too tightly, a missed section of diseased bowel, functional constipation, *neuronal intestinal dysplasia* (NID) (abnormal nerve cells near the segment of colon lacking nerve cells) or a hypertensive anal sphincter. Tests called colon and anorectal manometry can help determine which type of constipation the patient has.

The defecation cycle

Defecation in the adult human is a combination of both voluntary and involuntary processes (see Figure 37). The defecation cycle is defined as the interval of time between the completion of one bowel movement, and the completion of the following BM. At the start of the cycle, the rectum acts as a temporary compartment for the waste. Rectal walls expand as additional fecal matter enters the rectum. This increase in fecal material expands the rectum, and stimulates the stretch receptors in the wall of the rectum causing the relaxation of the internal anal sphincter and an initial contraction of the skeletal muscle of the external sphincter. The brain receives a signal from the relaxation of the internal anal sphincter indicating an urge to defecate.

The material in the rectum is often returned to the colon by reverse peristalsis if the defecation urge is ignored, where more water is absorbed. This temporarily decreases pressure and stretching within the rectum. The additional fecal material is then stored in the colon until the next peristaltic movement of the transverse and descending colon. If defecation is delayed for a prolonged period the fecal matter may harden and will result in constipation.

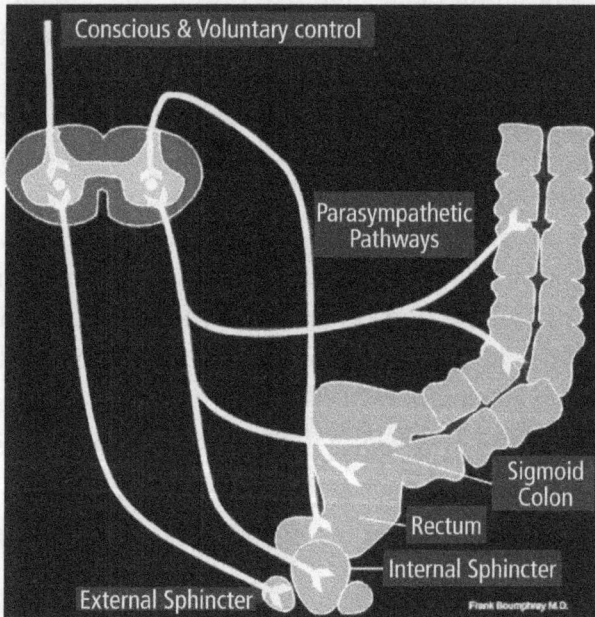

Figure 37. The defecation reflex by Dr. Frank Boumphreyfr, 2009.
Image reprinted with permission from Wikipedia Commons, 2011.

The final phase of the defecation cycle begins once the voluntary signal to defecate is sent back from the brain. Peristaltic waves cause the rectum to shorten and contract, pushing the waste out of the rectum and through the anal canal.

Functional constipation (encopresis)

Functional constipation happens most often following a painful bowel movement. Because of the pain, the child holds the stool and after a few days has a bigger, more painful bowel movement. Children with HD are more likely to develop functional constipation than other children because of the painful experiences they have had around the pelvic area.

Post pull-through diarrhea may cause such a bad diaper rash that the child has pain after a bowel movement. Dilatations are also very painful and frightening to the child and can cause them to hold in their stools. Dr. Paul Hyman (2005) found that these procedures can prevent the child from learning *pelvic floor* (muscles in pelvic area) control and may cause fear and retentive behavior. Because the child is afraid to have a bowel movement, the abdomen may swell and the doctor becomes concerned over ordering repeated enemas. In Dr. Hyman's opinion, these factors prevent the child from learning pelvic floor control.

After the danger of enterocolitis passes, Dr. Hyman recommends using an oral laxative like MiraLax® to melt away the stool mass. He believes that control must be given back to the child because the child learns to relax the pelvic floor only after associated fears have disappeared. In some cases of HD however, it is necessary for the child to have enemas on a daily basis. This is especially true if an oral laxative is ineffective.

Neuronal intestinal dysplasia (NID) or intestinal neuronal dysplasia (IND)

Intestinal neuronal dysplasia (IND) was first described by Meir-Ruge in 1971. Also referred to as neuronal intestinal dysplasia, it was classified as a colonic problem, although the disease can involve any portion of the GI tract. According to Dr. David Bliss of Emanuel Children's Hospital in Portland, Oregon, IND involves an abnormal number, type, size, and location of ganglion cells.

In IND, there can be areas that are skipped, where there are normal segments interspersed with segments that are affected. Most children complain of abdominal *distention* (gas) and have constipation. Some children with IND can develop enterocolitis, just like children with Hirschsprung's Disease. The symptoms of HD may mask those of the IND, so the diagnosis may not be made until the patient develops stooling problems after pull-through surgery (APSA, 2006).

The main difference between HD and IND is that the ganglion cells are present in IND but are virtually non-functioning. Another difference between Hirschsprung's Disease and IND is that the internal anal sphincter (IAS) relaxation reflex (also called the Anorectal Inhibitory Reflex (ARIR)) is absent or abnormal in Hirschsprung's Disease. The anus remains contracted in a normal person until a threshold pressure is reached in the anorectum (the anal canal and the first few centimeters of the rectum). This causes the involuntary sphincter muscles to relax, allowing for the passage of stool. This reflex is absent in classic HD therefore making it difficult for the person to have a bowel movement. In patients with IND, there can be an atypical ARIR as well (Tomita, Munakata, and Fukuzawa, 2000).

Around 10% of children with HD have abnormal nerve cells near the aganglionic segment. If a colon manometry is performed, it will show an abnormal result. There may be a segment with persistent pressure that fails to relax, a segment with no coordinated contractions, or a segment with no contractions. If the patient has a history of enterocolitis, anti-inflammatory drugs (*sulfasalizine*) or antibiotics (*metrinidazole* or *clarithromycin*) may help. When there is no history of enterocolitis, laxatives can help to maintain watery stools for life. Surgery is also an option if the neuropathy involves a longer colonic segment.

IND/NID can only be definitively diagnosed through a full-thickness biopsy of the bowel lining. IND/NID is often found in the transition zone between the healthy bowel and the HD diseased bowel. However, there are rare cases where IND is throughout the remainder of bowel (Busha, L., 2006). Currently, IND/NID is an incompletely understood entity that remains difficult for both clinicians and pathologists to precisely define (Curran, T., 2009).

Internal anal sphincter achalasia (IASA)/Hypertensive anal sphincter

Internal anal sphincter achalasia (IASA) is also referred to as ultra-short segment Hirschsprung's Disease (De Caluwe, Yoneda, Akl, and Puri, 2001) and hypertensive anal sphincter. IASA is similar to HD but the ganglion cells are present in the rectal biopsy. There are two sphincter muscles surrounding the anus: the external anal sphincter (EAS) and the internal anal sphincter (IAS). The internal anal sphincter muscle is involuntary, meaning that the person cannot control the contractions; the external anal sphincter is voluntarily controlled. Internal anal sphincter (IAS) achalasia is a disorder of defecation in which the IAS fails to relax. Some patients with HD also have IAS achalasia. An anal manometry will determine if the patient has IAS achalasia.

IAS achalasia is the least likely cause of constipation, affecting only 5% of children after surgery for HD (Hyman, 2005). In children with this disorder, pressures are so high in the sphincter that the stool cannot pass even when there is a contraction of the colon. Also called hypertensive anal sphincter (HAS), IAS achalasia is diagnosed by anal manometry while the child is asleep. Dr. Hyman of the University of Kansas Medical Center recommends a sphincterotomy or an anal myectomy instead of botulinum toxin injection in cases of HAS/IAS. Botulism injections often fail within a few months after treatment; however, incontinence can be a problem after a sphincterotomy or an anal myectomy.

Anal myectomy/sphincterotomy

Anorectal myectomy has been shown to provide long-term relief of chronic constipation in children with ultra-short Hirschsprung's Disease (Moore, Singaram, Eckhoff, Gammitz, and Starling, 1996). An anal myectomy involves cutting a 1 cm wide strip through the anal sphincter and muscles of the rectum to a variable length. This procedure is suggested for the treatment of ultra-short segment HD. A sphincterotomy is a procedure in which the internal anal sphincter muscle is cut.

Botox Injections

Botulinum toxin A (Botox®) is a neurotoxin produced by a bacterium called Clostridium botulinum. Botox temporarily blocks signals from the nerves to the muscles that are in constant contraction, causing the muscles it is injected into to relax. In Hirschsprung's patients, Botox can be injected into the internal anal sphincter (IAS). This causes the sphincter to relax and allow for a bowel movement. The Botox injections are done in the hospital under anesthesia by the child's surgeon.

The injection lasts for three to eight months and has been proven to be very effective in most patients (Ciamarra, Nurko, Barksdale, and Samuel, 2003). The child's surgeon can also suggest Botox injections during stool holding episodes. Stool holding is common during the potty-training years for every child but for children with HD, it can cause other complications such as severe constipation.

Hyperalgesia

Hyperalgesia is defined as a change in the child's perception that having a bowel movement hurts badly. In this disorder, abdominal pain may occur whenever the child senses the urge to defecate. The child then tightens the sphincter to avoid defecation. These children perceive these contractions as pain rather than as an urge to defecate, so the child no longer recognizes the feelings for a bowel movement.

Hyperalgesia is caused by changes in the pain nerves that run from the gut to the brain, and also the pain centers in the brain. Children with Hirschsprung's Disease who have had early life pain experiences such as surgery are at risk for developing hyperalgesia. There are drugs that can slowly reverse hyperalgesia as well as cognitive behavioral therapy (CBT) for school age children (Hyman, 2005).

Incontinence

Operations for Hirschsprung'S Disease can cause damage to the anal sphincters, which in turn can lead to fecal incontinence. Incontinence means that stool cannot be held in or that leaks may occur on passage of gas. Fecal incontinence can be divided into two categories: *real fecal incontinence* and *pseudoincontinence.*

Real fecal incontinence occurs when the muscles that control bowel movements (internal anal sphincter/external anal sphincter muscles) have been damaged. Nerves to these muscles can also be deficient or damaged so the child cannot distinguish between solid stools and gas. *Pseudoincontinence* occurs when the child behaves like he or she is fecally incontinent. Upon further investigation, however, it is discovered that the child is severely constipated and impacted. Once the impaction is treated with a gastrografin enema or with laxatives, the child becomes continent.

In one study conducted at the Institute of Child Health in London, it was found that long-term incontinence is common in patients with Hirschsprung's Disease regardless of the amount bowel affected. Incontinence affected a high proportion of the patients in the study, regardless of the extent of the disease. Another interesting find in this study was that those who were incontinent were no less well adjusted than those with bowel control. Compared with the surgeon's evaluation, the psychosocial interview revealed a higher proportion of incontinent patients among those with TCA. This suggests that postoperative functional problems may be under reported, especially to medical staff (Ludman, Spitz, Tsuji, and Pierro, 2002).

Enuresis (urinary incontinence)

Otherwise known as bed-wetting, enuresis is a loss of urine control specifically at night. Enuresis can be caused by surgery because the nerves to the bladder are located in the pelvic floor where Hirschsprung's surgery is performed. Although this rarely happens, these nerves can be damaged causing the patient to have problems with urination.

PREVENTING CONSTIPATION IN THE CHILD WITH HIRSCHSPRUNG'S DISEASE

IN SOME CHILDREN WITH HIRSCHSPRUNG'S DISEASE, keeping the bowels moving is a constant battle. Certain foods can cause constipation, while others can cause runny stools. Some ways to prevent constipation in the child with HD are listed below.

• Encourage the child to drink fluids

One job of the large intestine is to collect the water and salts the body needs. Because a child with HD has a shorter colon, less water is absorbed so Hirschsprung's patients need to drink more fluids than other children to compensate for this loss. Water is the best for rehydrating but Pedialyte® and Gatorade® can also help to restore the electrolytes in the body.

• Consume foods that are rich in fiber

The bulk in fruits, vegetables and whole grains such as wheat bread and bran cereals is beneficial. Prune and pear juices are rich in fiber as well. Diets that are high in fat, sugar, protein or dairy products may aggravate constipation. In general, goods that are from animal sources promote constipation, while foods from plant sources help with stooling.

• Take a fiber supplement like Benefiber®

Many times, children with HD don't seem to be constipated but they are. Fiber helps to hold the water in the colon so that defecation is easier and it keeps the child better hydrated. Fiber supplements can sometimes cause excessive gas; so watch the child closely for these symptoms.

• Keep a food and bowel movement diary

This will allow the parent to keep track of foods that should be avoided as well as foods that promote a healthy digestive system. Bowel movements can also be tracked, allowing the parents to work on a schedule for the child.

• Pay attention to the child's bowel habits

Encourage your child to go to the bathroom after each meal and whenever else he or she has the urge to go.

• Encourage daily exercise

Moving around is one of the best ways to get the digestive system moving. Exercise helps the digestive system flush waste from the body more quickly.

• Help the child relax

Keep a stack of magazines or books next to the toilet to give the child something to look at while having a bowel movement. Placing a footstool underneath the feet while the child is on the toilet will take pressure off of the pelvic bone and relax the muscles.

• Laxatives

The doctor may recommend a laxative or stool softener if improvements in the diet and toilet habits don't help with the child's constipation. Be sure to check with the doctor before giving any kind of laxative to a child.

• Keep the bottom clean

Clean the anal area with lukewarm water and a soft cloth or disposable wipes containing witch hazel. The witch hazel does not irritate the delicate skin surrounding the anus and the child can wipe him/herself during potty training. Soaps may irritate this sensitive area. Aquaphor® or Bag Balm is very helpful when the bottom is sore, even in older children.

• Talk with your child

Reassure your child that at some time in his/her life constipation will occur. Keep the lines of communication open even when the child becomes more modest.

HIRSCHSPRUNG'S DISEASE AND LAXATIVES

It is necessary for some children with Hirschsprung's Disease to be on a laxative after a pull-through operation. A laxative is used to help relieve constipation. There are five basic types of drugstore laxatives: bulk-forming laxatives, stool softening laxatives/emollients, lubricant laxatives, osmotic/saline laxatives, and stimulant laxatives (see Figure 38).

Possible side effects of stimulant laxatives

The nature of laxative dependence is a controversial issue. Laxative dependence may result from degeneration of the nerves in the intestines, causing a dulling affect on peristalsis, or may just be a psychological dependence. Naturally occurring stimulant laxatives are generally safe and gentle. A good example of a naturally occurring stimulant laxative is senna, which is derived from the senna leaf and pod. Senna has been used for centuries in China as a laxative. It is believed that senna works by irritating the intestinal wall, resulting in a bowel movement.

In the 1970's, *colonoscopy* (a procedure where the inside of the colon and rectum are examined) was developed as a routine diagnostic tool. It was discovered that many people had a black or dark brown intestinal wall. The condition was named *melanosis coli*, which is Latin for "black colon." Normally, the intestinal wall has a healthy pink appearance.

It was found that the darkened wall of the colon was associated with chronic use of a classification of laxatives known as *anthraquinone* laxatives. These laxatives are generally derived from plant sources. Examples of anthraquinone laxatives are senna, cascara sangria, buckthorn, and aloe. The anthraquinones are colorful, ranging from yellow to orange to red. Some doctors believe that the colon wall has simply been stained by the senna and view melanosis coli as a harmless and reversible condition. Other doctors believe that the dark colon color is a result of cellular damage in the wall of the colon (Dharmananda, 2009).

TYPES OF LAXATIVES	COMMON NAMES	HOW THEY WORK	SIDE EFFECTS
BULK-FORMING LAXATIVES (Effective within 1-3 days)	• *Bran* • *Fiberall* • *Hydrocil* • *Perdiem Fiber* • *Ultrafiber* • *Citrucel* • *Fibercon* • *Metamucil*	• Work by making your stools larger and heavier • Help to attract and trap water into their fiber structure. • Stimulates your colon to have a bowel movement. • Using laxatives that contain fiber is a natural way to stimulate your colon into action.	• Can cause gas and swelling in the abdomen resulting in an increase in flatulence. • Can also cause blockage in the bowel, so it is important to drink lots of water when taking bulk-forming laxatives. • Some bulk forming laxatives contain excess sugar and sodium. Read the label for these items, if you have high blood pressure, or are diabetic.
STIMULANT LAXATIVES (Effective within 6-24 hours)	• *ExLax* • *Glycerol suppositories* • *Senna/ Senekot* • *Syrup of figs*	• Work by increasing muscular contractions in the intestinal wall. • These contractions are responsible for moving waste along to the rectum for evacuation.	• Chemical dependency can occur when the product is taken daily or frequently over a long period of time. (The body will need to continue using it in order to have a normal bowel movement).
OSMOTIC/ SALINE LAXATIVES (Effective within 1-3 hours)	• *Lactulose syrup* • *MiraLax* • *Magnesium salts (Epsom salts)* • *Phosphate enemas* • *MicroLax enemas (sodium citrate)*	• Work by drawing more water into the bowel, making stools softer and easier to pass.	• Nausea, bloating, flatulence, and diarrhea. • In very rare cases, difficulty breathing, itching of the skin, hives, severe bloating, pain or distention of the stomach, and vomiting have been reported (MiraLax). • Can cause frequent bowel movements.
LUBRICANT LAXATIVES (Effective within 5-9 hours)	• *Mineral Oil* • *Kondremul*	• These simply make the stool slippery, so that it slides through the intestine more easily.	• Mineral oil may decrease the absorption of fat-soluble vitamins and some minerals. • Oil can leak into underwear
STOOL SOFTENING LAXATIVES/ EMOLLIENTS (Effective within 1-4 days)	• *Colace* • *Surfak Liqui-Gels*	• Stool softeners, called emollient laxatives, prevent hardening of the feces by adding moisture to the stool. • The active ingredient in most stool softeners is a medicine called docusate.	• Generally safe and well tolerated. • Do not combine with mineral oil, as stool softeners may increase the absorption and toxicity of mineral oil.

Figure 38. Comparing Laxatives. © 2010, Nicole Murphy.

PROBIOTICS AND HIRSCHSPRUNG'S DISEASE

PROBIOTICS ARE "FRIENDLY" BACTERIA that are found in a number of foods such as cheese and yogurt. In order to produce probiotics, the cheese and yogurt has to decompose or rot. This process is known as fermentation. When eaten, the bacteria colonize the gut and help to protect the body from illness. In the digestive tract, there exists a balance between healthy and harmful *microflora* (bacteria). When a person is healthy, over 100 trillion microorganisms flourish in the intestinal tract (Barron, 1999).

The digestive tract is actually a complex ecosystem that is responsible for producing enzymes to digest and absorb nutrients and rid the body of harmful toxins. Although some bacteria can harm us, certain species of bacteria are essential for maintaining good health. These "good microbes" improve digestive function and also keep the "bad microbes" at bay.

Antibiotics, although necessary for killing the bad microbes to fight disease, also kill the good microbes in the intestines. Antibiotics are creating "super germs" that are drug resistant and impossible to restrain. Eliminating all of the good microbes from our body results in a weaker immune system causing problems like increased allergies and asthma. According to a University of Nebraska Medical Center study, nearly 30 percent of children given antibiotics suffer from diarrhea as a result (Siegel-Maier, 2007).

Yogurt containing Lactobacillus acidophilus is often recommended by practitioners to help reduce the side effects of oral antibiotic therapy in patients. In one study, it was found that 89% of patients complaining of diarrhea during a round of oral antibiotics improved significantly when given Lactobacillus acidophilus (J Otolaryngol,

1995). Probiotic microbes do not cause disease and they taste good so there is no such thing as having too many of them (Huffnagle, 2006).

Recently, there have been many studies done which show that probiotics help improve the function of the gut by eliminating harmful bacteria in children with motility issues like Hirschsprung's Disease. Lactobacillus acidophilus has also been shown to reduce cancer causing agents in the gut as well as decreasing cholesterol levels in most patients (Crit Rev Microbiol, 1995). Lactobacillus GG has been shown to alleviate intestinal inflammation as well as eczema and food allergies (J Allergy Clin Immunol, 1997). Bifidobacteria increases *antibodies* (proteins that fight infection) secreted in the body, resulting in increased resistance against infections of the intestinal tract (*Int J Food Microbiol.*, 1998).

Lactobacillus acidophilus is helpful in preventing vaginal yeast infections. Bifidobacterium, protect us from *carcinogens* (cancer causing agents) created during the process of cooking food. Unfortunately, as the human body ages, the levels of beneficial bacteria decline dramatically.

Some reasons for this include:
- Use of anti-inflammatory drugs such as Advil, Motrin, Midol, etc. is destructive to intestinal flora.
- Chlorine in drinking water kills the bacteria in the water but also the beneficial bacteria in the intestinal tract.
- All meat, chicken and dairy that we eat (other than organic) contain antibiotics, which destroy all of the beneficial bacteria living in the gut.
- Cigarettes, alcohol and stress decrease healthy bacteria levels.
- Antibiotics are the number one culprits in the overgrowth of harmful *pathogens* (disease-causing organisms) in the intestinal tract. These pathogens may be the cause of many autoimmune disorders and certain types of cancer.

An allergy is a misguided reaction to a foreign substance (cow's milk, for example) by the immune system. Eosinophils are a type of white blood cell that is released during an allergic reaction. These cells secrete an anti-inflammatory protein called *histamine*. People with allergies have a high number of eosinophils in their system. The probiotic Lactobacillus GG has anti-inflammatory capabilities by preventing the production of eosinophils. In one study, it was found that probiotic bacteria helped to alleviate intestinal inflammation in patients with food and skin allergies (J Allergy Clin Immunol, 1997).

Other benefits of a healthy intestinal tract (one that contains enough probiotics) include:

- Lowered cholesterol levels
- Inhibition of cancer
- Protection against food poisoning
- Protection against stomach ulcers
- Protection against lactose intolerance
- Enhanced immunity
- Protection against many harmful bacteria, viruses, and fungi
- Protection against vaginal yeast infections
- Prevention and correction of constipation and diarrhea and other digestive tract dysfunctions.
- Improvement of health and appearance of the skin
- Better nutrition from improved absorption of vitamins.

A probiotic formula based on L. acidophilus and bifidobacteria will maintain a healthy intestinal tract. L. acidophilus resides in the small intestine and produces antimicrobial compounds. These compounds can inhibit the growth and toxin producing capabilities of many disease-causing organisms as well as inhibiting carcinogenic substances and reducing tumor growth.

Bifidobacteria lives mainly in the large intestine and prevents chronic degenerative diseases. These bacteria consume old fecal matter, remove cancer-forming enzymes and protect against the formation of liver, colon, and mammary gland tumors. Other bacteria that are extremely beneficial are:

- *L. salivarius* – Helps to digest foods and repair the intestinal tract.

• *L. rhamnosus* – A powerful immune stimulator that can increase circulating antibody levels by six to eight times.

• *L. plantarum* – Can eliminate thousands of species of bad bacteria like E-coli.

There are many probiotics on the market. Some products that contain probiotics and are easy for children to eat are Kieffer® fruit smoothies and Dannon® yogurt. It is important to be sure that the probiotic contains active cultures like L. burglaricus, S. thermophilus, and Bifidobacterium. A good probiotic formula will also contain fructooligosaccharides (a class of non-digestible sugars that occur naturally in some plants, which help promote the growth of the beneficial bacteria). When the fructooligosaccharides reach the colon, they are used by the good bacteria for growth and multiplication.

When beginning a probiotic supplement, it is very important to start slowly. As the bad bacteria begin to die off, gas, stomach rumblings, and cramping for up to three weeks can occur (Barron, 1999). It is especially important for children with Hirschsprung's Disease to begin slowly so as not to cause further problems.

HIRSCHSPRUNG'S DISEASE AND DECREASED IMMUNITY

IT IS IMPORTANT TO REMEMBER that the entire digestive tract is lined with a mucous membrane. This membrane protects the underlying tissues and also allows for the absorption of nutrients from digested food in the intestine. In order to function properly in absorbing nutrients, the membrane must be thin and moist. The membrane also serves to protect the intestines from viruses and harmful bacteria.

Patients with Hirschsprung's Disease can have an abnormal mucous composition in the gut, particularly those who are more susceptible to enterocolitis (Akkary, Sahwy, Kandil, and Hamdy, 1981). This finding is important because contained in the mucous of the gut are *antibodies* (a type of immunoglobin) which help to destroy *viruses* and *bacteria* (small organisms that can be harmful). Akkary did not notice a difference in the secretion of mucous from the intestines but did notice that there was an increase in the sulphated mucins in the gut of HD patients. This difference was especially noticeable in patients who had enterocolitis.

More recent studies have shown that the turnover of mucins produced by patients with HD is slower than control patients, suggesting that there is an abnormal mucous defense barrier that contributes to HAEC (Aslam, Spicer, and Corfield, 1997). Many scientists feel that this and could be the reason HD patients seem to be more affected by the common stomach flu. However, this theory has yet to be proven.

T-lymphocytes are white blood cells that help our bodies to battle infection. These cells are located in various parts of the body and their mission is to find and destroy virus-infected cells. An analysis of white blood cell counts of infants with HAEC has shown that they have lower counts and a decreased white blood cell function when compared to other patients (Wilson-Storey & Scobie, 1989).

Immunoglobins are a type of protein called an antibody. In response to unwanted viruses or bacteria, the body makes these antibodies. When an *antigen* (foreign invader) is found, the antibodies attack, preventing the virus or bacteria from binding to the GI tract. Because the antigen cannot bind to the GI tract, it cannot cause illness.

Immunoglobin A (IgA) protects the mucous membranes of the body and is found in large quantities in the intestinal tract. One study found that immunoglobins were not released into the *lumen* (inner wall of the intestines), suggesting that there may be a defect in the release of these substances in the HD patient (Wilson-Storey et al., 1989). In one study of the *lamina propria* (the layer of the mucous membrane that contains the blood vessels, lymph nodes and small glands), IgA levels were lower in HD patients, and even lower levels were found in patients with HAEC (Turnock, Spitz, Strobel, 1992). It was discovered by Imanmura, Pur, O'Brian, and Reein (1989) that Nitric oxide levels are decreased in the aganglionic portion of HD patients. A decline in the production of nitric oxide may result in a deficient barrier against disease causing organisms in patients with Hirschsprung's Disease.

HIRSCHSPRUNG'S DISEASE AND GASTROENTERITIS

GASTROENTERITIS IS A GENERAL TERM for infection or irritation of the digestive tract, mainly the stomach and intestines. Many things (including viruses, bacteria, and parasites) can cause it. Gastroenteritis is generally called the stomach flu, but is not truly *influenza* (a respiratory illness). Major symptoms are nausea, vomiting, diarrhea, and abdominal cramps. A fever, general aches, and weakness may also be symptoms. Gastroenteritis usually lasts around three days. Adults can usually recover without any complications but children, the elderly, and anyone with other underlying disease are more likely to have complications such as dehydration (*Encyclopedia of Medicine, 2007*).

Gastroenteritis vs. enterocolitis

After a pull-through operation, it is sometimes difficult to tell the difference between gastroenteritis and enterocolitis. A case of enterocolitis can be brought on by gastroenteritis. The only way to be certain about what is causing the illness is to run blood and fecal tests. The doctor will then be able to determine how the patient with HD should be treated.

Rotavirus

Many different viruses can cause gastroenteritis and children can have an array of symptoms. Typically, children are more susceptible to rotaviruses. Rotavirus causes fever, vomiting, and watery diarrhea. Children can have a lot of watery diarrhea and can be sick with rotavirus for up to nine days. Rotavirus is highly contagious and is typically spread by touching contaminated surfaces and then touching the mouth and ingesting the germs (fecal oral route) (RotavirusInfo.com,

2007). This virus can be especially dangerous for the child with Hirschsprung's Disease.

Dehydration

During a bout of gastroenteritis, a child who has Hirschsprung's Disease may not be able to keep enough fluids in the body to stay hydrated. The main function of the colon is to absorb water and *electrolytes* (salts and minerals). A severe bout of diarrhea and vomiting may deplete the water and electrolytes in the body so quickly that the child cannot keep up, especially if the child has had some or the entire colon removed. In some cases, *IV therapy* (replacing fluids and electrolytes through an IV) may be necessary to keep the child hydrated during an illness of this nature.

Some symptoms of dehydration are no urine in the diaper, no tears when crying, a dry mouth, sunken eyes and *fontanels* (soft spot) in babies, and extreme thirst in older children (*Encyclopedia of Medicine*, 2007). Dehydration can cause the electrolytes in the body to become unbalanced, leading to heart arrhythmia and even death. (RotavirusInfo.com, 2007).

GENETICS AND HIRSCHSPRUNG'S DISEASE

CHROMOSOMES ARE THREAD-LIKE STRUCTURES that contain the information of heredity for living organisms (see Figure 39). They are found in the nucleus of the cell. Each human body cell has 46 chromosomes made up of 22 pairs of *autosomes* (all chromosomes except for the sex chromosomes) and one pair of *sex chromosomes* (XX = female or XY = male). The number of chromosomes in every species varies greatly. These chromosomes carry all of the genetic information for that individual.

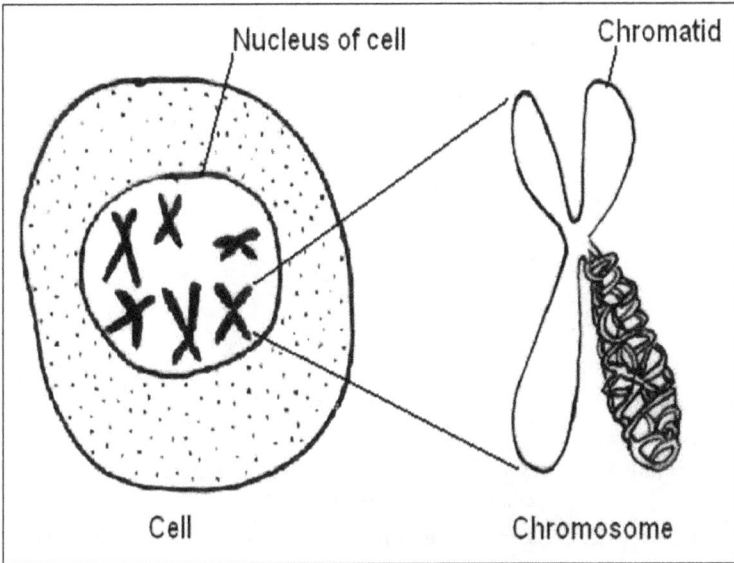

Figure 39. Picture of human chromosome.
Image reprinted with permission from Wikimedia Commons, 2011.

Sex chromosomes

Males have one X chromosome and one Y chromosome and females have two X chromosomes. Contained in the sperm cell is either an X chromosome or a Y chromosome. When the sperm cell combines with the woman's egg cell, which always is X, the sex of the offspring is decided (see Figure 40). For example, if an X sperm fertilizes an egg, the offspring will be XX or female. If a Y sperms fertilizes an egg, the offspring will be XY or male.

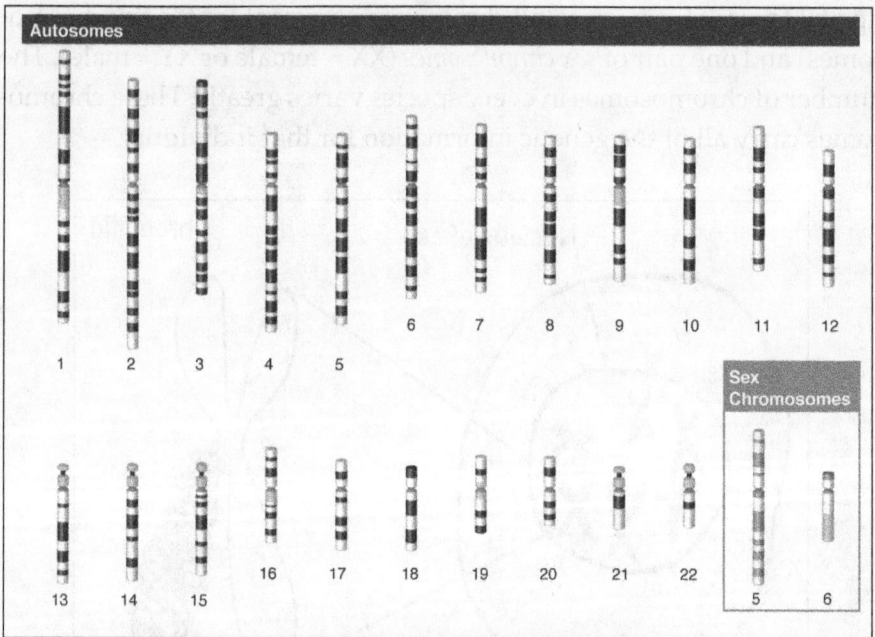

Figure 40. 22 pairs of human chromosomes and the 23rd pair of sex chromosomes (human male).

Image reprinted with permission from Wikimedia Commons, 2011.

Genes

A gene is a region on the chromosome that passes on characteristics and tendencies from parent to offspring, and each has a place on a specific chromosome (see Figure 41). The Danish geneticist Wilhelm Johannsen, in 1909, described a gene in terms of a characteristic of an individual, like brown or blue eyes (*World of Science*, 2005).

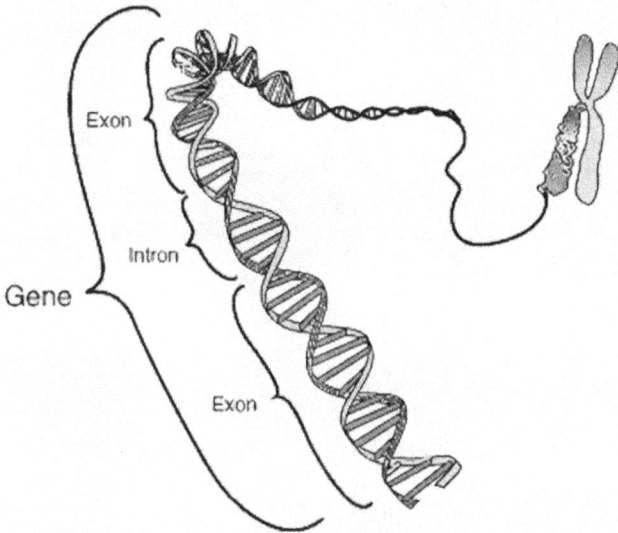

Figure 41. Chromosome showing regions called "genes."
Image reprinted with permission from Wikimedia Commons, 2011.

Mendelian genetics

In 1865, Gregor Mendel published a paper in which he described the reproduction of peas. He noted the inherited traits of each generation and called these traits dominant and recessive characteristics. In fact, Mendel had discovered genes. Mendel also discovered that genes also have *alleles* (or variations), like BB for brown eyes or bb for blue eyes. Some of these alleles show dominance and cover the other alleles known as recessive (see Figure 42).

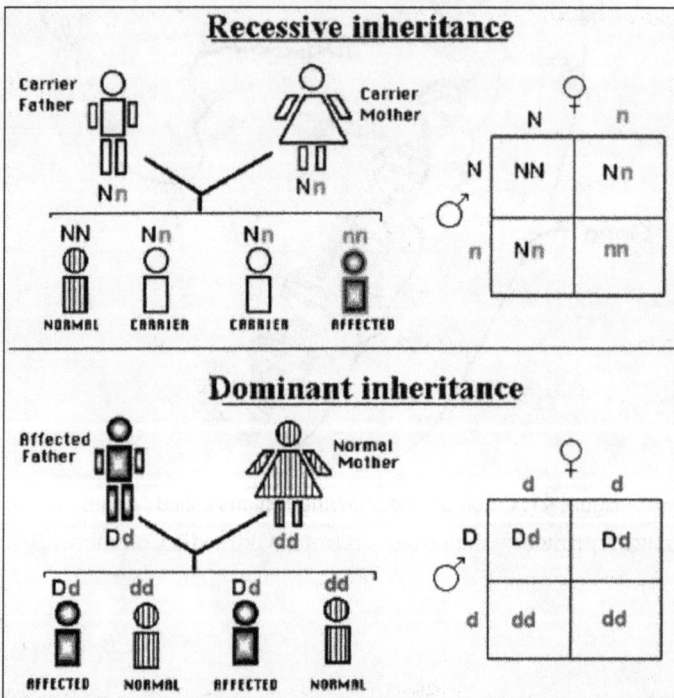

Figure 42. Diagram showing recessive and dominant inheritance patterns.
Image courtesy of the National Human Genome Research Institute, www.genome.gov, 2010.

DNA

Today, a gene is defined as a segment of DNA (Deoxyribonucleic Acid). Each chromosome consists of a DNA molecule and the genes are lined up along the chromosome, like beads on a string. These genes carry the secrets of life. DNA has all of the information needed to build, control and maintain a living organism. J.D. Watson and F.C. Crick, in 1953, discovered that DNA is arranged in a *double helix* (ladder-shaped) fashion (see Figure 43).

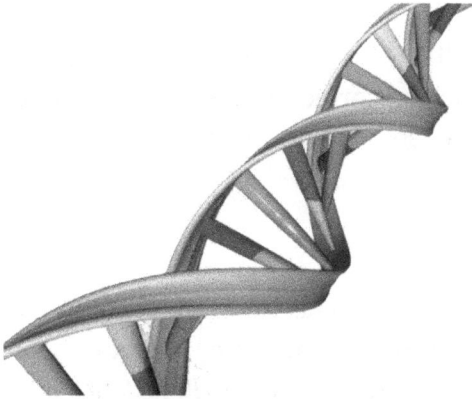

Figure 43. Double helix structure of a DNA molecule.
Image courtesy of the National Human Genome Research Institute, www.genome.gov, 2005.

Protein synthesis

The rungs of the ladder in the DNA molecule are made of subunits called adenine, guanine, thymine, and cytosine. Adenine binds with thymine: guanine binds with cytosine. The hereditary characteristics of living organisms are determined by the sequencing of these subunits or bases. If TGC (Thymine, Guanine, and Cytosine) were represented, its complimentary bases would be ACG, causing the amino acid tyrosine to be produced. This base triplet is called a *codon*, or a code word for a specific amino acid. After many amino acids are linked together, a protein is formed.

Humans have around 20,000 genes (*World of Science*, 2005). Genes determine the proteins that are made in each cell. Structural proteins such as collagen and keratin provide strength to connective tissues like tendons and ligaments. *Enzymes* (which aid in digestion), *antibodies* (which protect us from illness), and cell receptors are all types of proteins.

Mutations

A genetic disorder is a disease caused by a change in the DNA sequence. These changes are also called mutations and can be caused by a mistake in the cell or by outside influences like radiation or chemicals. Any change in the correct base sequences can cause a different protein to be made, sometimes causing a devastating effect on the organism.

Types of genetic disorders

The National Human Genome Research Institute states that genetic disorders can be grouped into three categories: single gene disorders, chromosome disorders, and *multi-factorial inheritance disorders* (Hirschsprung's Disease).

1. *Single gene disorders.* Single gene disorders are caused by a mistake in a single gene. The mutation can be on one or both chromosomes of a pair. Sickle cell anemia, cystic fibrosis, and Fragile X disease are examples of single gene disorders.

2. *Chromosome disorders.* Chromosome disorders result from an abnormal number of chromosomes, leading to too many or too few copies of a set of genes. An extra copy of a chromosome causes Down syndrome. As discussed in the Appendix, children with this syndrome have three of the 21st chromosome instead of only two. No individual gene is abnormal but the extra chromosome causes many problems.

3. Multi-factorial inheritance disorders. Multi-factorial disorders are caused by a combination of small variations in genes, often interacting with environmental factors. Alzheimer's disease, heart disease, most cancers, and Hirschsprung's Disease are all examples of these types of genetic disorders.

According to Julie Albertus of Johns Hopkins University, the majority of people with HD (90%) have no family history. However, in families where there are several cases, it is not uncommon for the disease to skip generations. There may be people in a family who carry these "susceptibility genes"; when they are combined with other "susceptibility genes," Hirschsprung's Disease can be the result.

So far, eight genes have been identified in HD but changes in other unknown genes exist. Genes on Chromosomes 1, 2, 3, 5, 10, 13, 19, and 20, have all been linked to Hirschsprung's Disease (see Figure 44). The RET gene, located on Chromosome 10, is the major cause of Hirschsprung's Disease. Other genes responsible for HD are EDNRB (chromosome 13), GDNF (chromosome 5), ECE1 (chromosome 1), NRTN (chromosome 19), EDN3 (chromosome 20), SOX10 (chromosome 22), and SIP1 (chromosome 2) (PubMed Central, 2005).

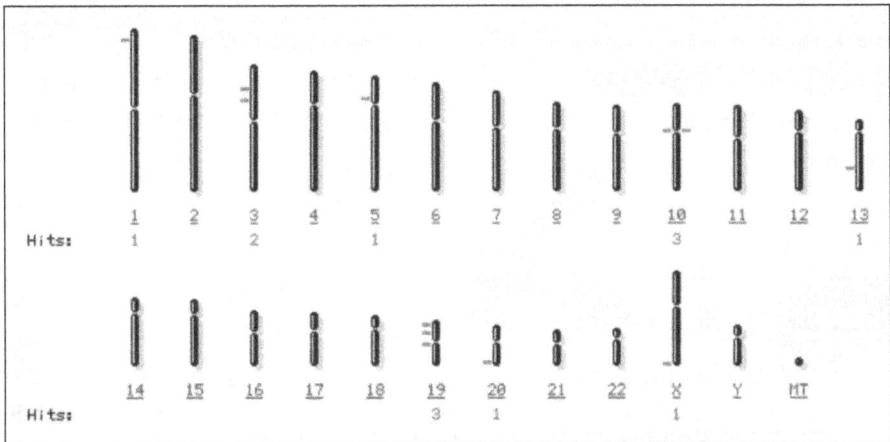

Figure 44. Genes on human chromosomes that cause Hirschsprung's Disease.
The shaded lines denote the regions on the genes that can interact with other genes to cause HD.

Image courtesy of the National Human Genome Research Institute,
www.genome.gov, 2010.

When a child has long-segment HD, it is more likely that multiple family members will also be affected. Also, the male-to-female ratio of 4:1 is decreased so that there is almost an equal number of males and females with LSHD. The inheritance pattern for this type of HD is more likely to be a single mutation in the RET gene (autosomal dominant). For children with shorter segments involved, the inheritance pattern is autosomal recessive. The likelihood of finding a mutation is less than 50% and may be as low as 10%. There is, however, a greater chance of finding a mutation if there is a family history and or Long-segment/Total colonic HD (Albertus, 2005).

RET gene

Dr. Bob Sawin of Seattle's Children's Hospital states that the RET gene is the most important gene when looking at the genetic cause of HD. RET is also associated with thyroid cancer and neuroblastoma. Both of these disorders have also been observed in Hirschsprung's patients with greater frequency than in the general population (Sawin, 2005).

Mutations in the RET gene cause it to become inactive. RET occurs in the neural crest stem cells 100 times more frequently than in other fetal cells. Three other genes—Sox 10, GFR alpha-1, and endothelin receptor type B (EDNRB)—were also found to be at higher levels (Morrison, 2003). In 2002, other scientists found that two mutated genes must interact to cause Hirschsprung's Disease. RET was found on chromosome 10, but must interact with EDNRB, a gene on chromosome 13, to cause HD in most cases. The specific origins of HD are still not completely understood.

Complexity of Hirschsprung's Disease

70% of Hirschsprung's Disease cases are isolated, meaning that no one else in the family has the disease (Nichols, 2010). There are around 8 to 10 genes associated with HD and greater than 100 mutations. All are caused by different interactions of the above genes, which makes HD a very complex disease. According to geneticists at Johns Hopkins

School of Medicine, the percent risk for families depends on several factors (see Figure 45).

% Risk to relatives	Rectosigmoid (short-segment)		Colonic-segment (descending colon)		Long-segment & Total colonic HD	
	Male	Female	Male	Female	Male	Female
Siblings of affected males	4-5%	1%	9-10%	7%	9-12%	7-9%
Siblings of affected females	5-6%	1-2%	12-13%	10%	21-24%	17-19%
Offspring of affected males	0-1%	<1%	10-11%	8-9%	16-19%	21-24%
Offspring of affected females	0-1%	<1%	14-15%	11%	27-29%	21-22%

Figure 45. Inheritance patterns in Hirschsprung's Disease.
*For example, if you have a son with long-segment HD, and your next child is a girl, her chance to have HD is 7-9%. Your son's chance to have a son with HD is 16-19%. *

Image reprinted with permission from Badner et al. *Am. J. Hum. Genet.* 1990.
http://www.hopkinsmed.org
geneticmedicine/clinicalResources/Hirschsprung/Home-Hirschsprung.html

HIRSCHSPRUNG'S DISEASE AND MY SON KELLEN

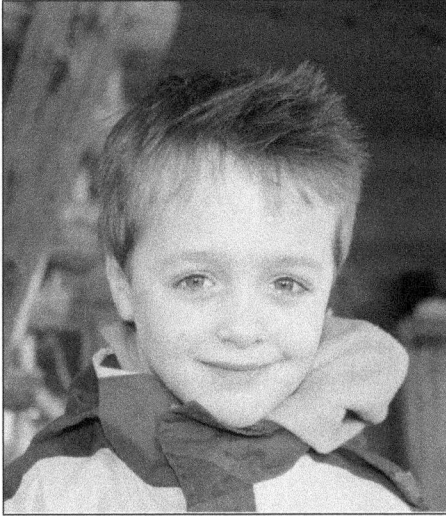

Fig. 46 Kellen, age 7.

BECAUSE EVERY CHILD with Hirschsprung's Disease is different, it is ultimately up to the parent to figure out what works best for their son or daughter. Keeping a food and pooping diary helps the parent remember the little details. It may also be a good idea to meet with a nutritionist to come up with a diet plan for your child. A nutritionist can teach parents which foods are constipating and which ones can cause loose stools. Although Kellen is now seven years old, my husband Bryan and I are still learning how to cope with his disease. In the following paragraphs, I have made some suggestions on foods to avoid, barrier ointments, constipation, potty training, exercise, stomach flu, and probiotics.

Foods to avoid

We have learned that there are certain foods Kellen cannot have. Popcorn, nuts, beans, and corn can cause him to have pain during a bowel movement (BM). Too many vegetables and fruits in one day give him diarrhea and a very red bottom. We know now when he is holding his stool in because his tummy makes very loud grumbling noises. Immediately, we put him on the toilet and he proceeds to let it all out. He has never had a loud belly and not had to go to the bathroom.

When Kellen has a red bottom he is afraid to poop because it hurts. He will hold it in and cry for fear of pain upon pooping (hyperalgesia). This turns into a vicious cycle that is hard to break. He can eat fruits and veggies, but not in large quantities. We have found that pear actually helps him to have more regular bowel movements and so we try to give him some at least once a day. After seven years, he is *finally* beginning to listen to his body and will go sit on the potty when he has the urge.

Barrier ointments

For the red bottom, we use Aquaphor® ointment. It seems to work the best because it forms a barrier on the skin. In the evening, Bryan and I goop large amounts of Aquaphor® on his bottom and put his pull-up on to protect the skin in case of a bowel movement in the middle of the night. Other moms I have spoken with swear by ILEX® cream (a skin protectant paste) for the bad diaper rashes babies can have after a pull-through operation.

Dealing with constipation

Constipation is defined as bowel movements that are infrequent and/or hard to pass (Wikipedia, 2011). Constipation is a common cause of painful defecation. Severe constipation includes failure to pass stools or gas and fecal impaction. Kellen's pediatrician recommended that his stools ideally have the texture of soft serve ice cream. This consistency makes it the easiest for a child to have a successful bowel movement.

During my research on constipation, I came across the **Bristol Stool Chart** (see Figure 47) and have used it as a guide in determining whether or not Kellen is constipated. The **Bristol Stool Chart** (see Figure 47) classifies the form of human feces into seven categories. The form of the stool depends on the time it spends in the colon. Types 1 and 2 indicate constipation, with 3 and 4 being the "ideal stools" especially the latter, as they are the easiest to defecate, and 5 to 7 tending towards diarrhea (Lewis & Heaton, 1997).

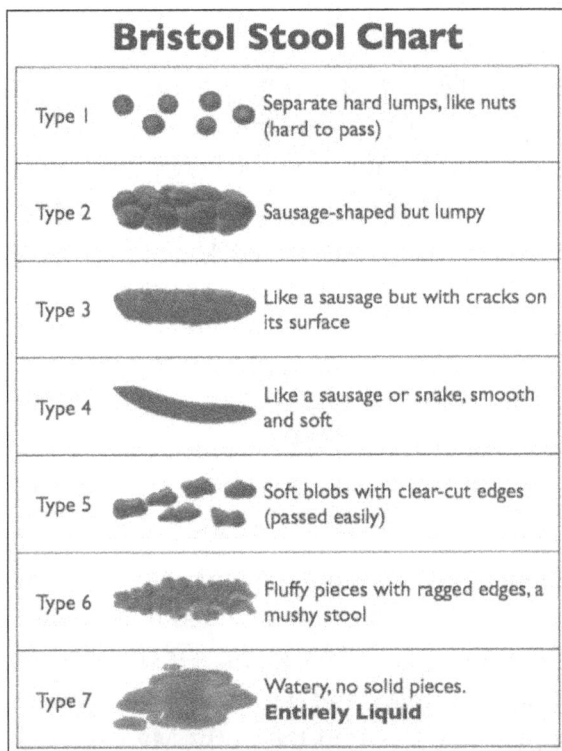

Bristol Stool Chart

Type 1	Separate hard lumps, like nuts (hard to pass)
Type 2	Sausage-shaped but lumpy
Type 3	Like a sausage but with cracks on its surface
Type 4	Like a sausage or snake, smooth and soft
Type 5	Soft blobs with clear-cut edges (passed easily)
Type 6	Fluffy pieces with ragged edges, a mushy stool
Type 7	Watery, no solid pieces. **Entirely Liquid**

Figure 47. Bristol Stool Chart.
Image reprinted with permission from Wikimedia Commons, 2011.

After the second operation, Bryan and I realized that Kellen's problems were mostly due to constipation. His pediatrician recommended Miralax®, a stool softener and mild laxative. We started giving Kellen small doses of Miralax® every day on a sort of sliding scale. If he ate a lot of fruits and veggies, he got less Miralax® and if he ate more constipating foods, he got more Miralax®.

The only problem we found with this method was that he constantly had smears of feces in his underwear. We figured out that this meant he was still constipated so recently, we have been giving him a capful of Miralax® every day. The problem with this was that he constantly had to go to the bathroom. I felt like I could never leave my house!

Bryan and I decided to give the stimulant laxative ex-lax® a try during the potty-training phase in order to give Kellen more sensation that he had to "go." We would give him ½ of a chocolate chewable at night with one fiber pill and it worked like a charm. We made sure to have him drink a glass of water with the fiber pill as it can cause constipation on its own. Kellen would have a BM every morning and would go once or twice more during the day. Using the stronger stimulant laxative helped Kellen realize that he needed time on the potty. Once he learned to listen to his body, we took him off of the ex-lax® and started him back on the Miralax® and fiber. Now, we give him his nightly drink of one Tbsp Metamucil®, and one capful of Miralax®. This seems to be the perfect concoction for Kellen.

Potty-training

The main difference between potty-training girls and boys is that boys don't seem to care if they have wet or soiled underpants. A few of my friends whose sons don't have HD, still soil their underpants from time to time. Kellen loves to play and sometimes just goes in his pants to avoid quitting playtime to sit on the potty. My two girls on the other hand, were much more concerned about having excrement in their underwear.

Bryan and I started potty-training Kellen at about three and a half years of age. We bought about thirty pairs of underpants because we knew we would be changing a lot of them. When we went out in public, Kellen would wear a pull-up and while we were at home, he wore underpants. Sometimes, I put a mini-pad in the back part of his underwear to prevent soiling in case of an accident.

In order to get him to sit on the potty for a longer period of time, we set up a small MP3 video player in his bathroom and played his favorite videos while he was on the toilet. The MP3 player helped Kellen to relax during a BM so could more easily have a bowel movement.

Once he learned how to settle down during a BM, we took away the video player and substituted it with a timer (kitchen timers work great). We set the timer for five minutes and when it went off, he knew he was finished. Kellen was then asked to push a few more times to completely empty his rectum before getting off of the potty. We randomly chose five minutes and it happened to work for Kellen, however, the time it takes to complete a BM will vary for every child.

Rewarding Kellen for going to the bathroom was a priority as well. We started giving him an incentive by keeping a bowl of skittles in the bathroom. If he went to the bathroom on his own and washed his hands, he got to pick one skittle as a reward. Unfortunately, the novelty of the skittles wore off after a few months. Bryan and I also tried letting him pick a toy (from the $$ store) out of a bag if he could keep his underwear/pull-up clean for a period of time. Now, we just use verbal praise when he keeps himself clean.

Now, he plays his Leapster™ while on the potty. This offers a distraction for him and allows him to sit there a little longer. Kellen still tries to avoid sitting on the potty but is learning that it is something everyone has to do.

It has been a very slow process but now at age seven, he is finally potty-trained during the day (we are still working on nights). The key for Kellen was going to school all day and having to learn to be more responsible for his own bathroom time. He is on a 504 plan (these plans have different names depending on where you live) through his school, where a staff member walks him down to the main office every day after lunch to sit on the toilet. He has a change of underpants and jeans in "his" bathroom and is reminded by the office ladies to spend some time on the potty.

We have learned that Kellen needs to have a BM about three times a day—especially after meals. It is important that your child have a private place to use the bathroom at school if this is embarrassing for him/her. Remember that it can take years for the colon to relearn it's job and every child is different.

Kellen generally has to go to the bathroom after he eats so we try not to let him snack frequently as this causes him to have to go to the bathroom more often. We have learned that three meals a day and a snack in the afternoon work the best for him. He is also required to sit on the potty after breakfast, lunch, and dinner. Unless we hear his stomach rumbling, we don't pressure him to use the bathroom more than this.

Since we have started using the Miralax® and Metamucil® combination, Kellen doesn't constantly have small amounts of poop on his bottom. As a result, the skin around his anus is not red or bleeding anymore. Lately, we have been using disposable wet wipes that he can wipe himself with after a bowel movement. I have him do the first few wipes with toilet paper, and then he has to use the wet wipe to get the stool off of his bottom. I do a final check myself with a wet wipe after he has finished. Using this method has spared his bottom that nasty rash we are all so used to.

Exercise

Exercise is also very important for Kellen because it keeps his bowels moving. On days when the weather is bad and we aren't outside, he tends to get more constipated. When he is outside playing, he poops more easily and more frequently.

Exercise helps to prevent constipation by decreasing the time it takes food to move through the large intestine, thus limiting the amount of water absorbed from the stool into your body. Hard, dry stools are harder to pass. Aerobic exercises like walking or running, accelerate breathing and heart rate. This stimulates the natural contraction of intestinal muscles, which move stools quickly out of the body.

Gastroenteritis

A bout of *gastroenteritis* (stomach flu) can land Kellen in the hospital. Due to a lowered immune response in the mucous lining of the intestines in some children with HD, the stomach flu can cause a lot of problems for them. When he was younger, Kellen had to have IV therapy for a few days in the hospital. We had to do irrigations during the flu to help keep things moving. As he has gotten older, we have been able to quit doing the irrigations.

During our last stay in the hospital, an ER doctor suggested trying a medication called *Zofran*™ (Also called Ondansetron, Zofran™ is a drug prescribed for children undergoing chemotherapy and is used to relieve nausea). I call it the "magic pill" because the last few times Kellen had gastroenteritis, it prevented him from vomiting and ultimately going into the hospital.

I asked his pediatrician about the dangers of preventing vomiting in a child with gastroenteritis and he told me that most of the virus is shed in the feces. So if fluid loss can be prevented, the child with Hirschsprung's Disease may not have to be hospitalized for dehydration. Although the medication is expensive, it does not hold a candle to the cost of a few days in the hospital.

I still keep his irrigation tube and saline solution handy just in case he needs help with pooping during an illness. It has been four years since our last hospital stay. He is getting stronger the older he gets. Kellen now weighs 51 lbs. and is a happy healthy seven-year-old. He is right on track for growth and development and is actually big for his age. Because he has more frequent bowel movements than the average child, we have to be more aware of where the bathrooms are in public places.

Probiotics

Kellen eats one vanilla Dannon® yogurt a day with probiotics in it. This has really helped him, especially during a course of antibiotics. The probiotics have helped him to maintain a healthy intestinal tract. He seems to have had a much better winter than usual since we started giving him the yogurt.

What I have learned from Hirschsprung's Disease

This disease has taught me to be patient and understanding. It has given me a new perspective on life. I have learned to take one day at a time and to not worry as much about the small things. I have made many new friends who are also living with HD. Many times I was so scared—not knowing when to do an irrigation, or when to take Kellen to the ER. I felt so alone during this time because I didn't know anyone else in my small town that had a child with HD. To make matters worse, we lived three hours away from his surgeons.

One of the positive things that came out of my experience with Hirschsprung's Disease is that I learned that I could write a book—something I never thought about doing before this rare disease entered into my life. I truly think things happen for a reason. Kellen is a gift from God. He has taught me many things that I wouldn't have learned without him. So I guess in a strange way, I am thankful that we went through this experience together. It has truly made our bond as mother and son stronger and very special.

APPENDIX

In most cases, Hirschsprung's Disease is easily managed after surgery; however, more acute forms of HD generally require additional care. I have included this appendix for readers who may need more information on Hirschsprung associated syndromes, different types of testing, as well as information on how to care for a patient with a more extensive form of Hirschsprung's Disease.

Remember that the care instructions (TPN, Stoma, and Mickey Button) are suggestions only. TPN, Stoma, and Mickey Button guidelines are standardized in hospitals that provide this service, so be sure to check with your child's doctor and nurses before implementing any of these techniques. The following topics will be discussed in this appendix:

- Guidelines for caring for your ill child
- Further testing (colon manometry and anal manometry)
- Care tips (stoma care, mickey button care, and TPN line care)
- Syndromes associated with Hirschsprung's Disease
  (Down syndrome,
  Shah-Waardenberg syndrome,
  Haddad syndrome,
  Mowat-Wilson syndrome,
  Goldberg-Shprintzen syndrome,
  Cartilage-hair hypoplasia syndrome,
  Bardet-Biedle syndrome, and
  Smith-Lemli-Opitz syndrome).
- Bowel management (Dr. Marc Levitt)

GUIDELINES FOR CARING FOR YOUR ILL CHILD

Interacting effectively with doctors, nurses, and medical staff

- The parents and the medical staff are a *team* working towards a common goal: the health of your child.
- The parents are a vital member of the team and have a right to medical information about the child.
- Communicate clearly with your doctors about the information you want or need in order to feel comfortable with the treatment plan. I found it helpful to carry a notebook with me so that I could take notes while the doctor spoke. Then if I had any questions later, I could refer back to my notes.
- If you don't understand something, be sure to clarify with the doctors. Keep asking until you feel comfortable with the explanations. You won't be able to make informed decisions unless you understand the plan of action.
- The pharmacist is a part of the medical team and has much knowledge about the medications given to your child. He or she knows the possible drug interactions as well as current research on various drugs. I always picked the pharmacists brain on the medications prescribed for Kellen.
- Nurses are wonderful resources and can serve as an advocate for your child. Their role is to help the patient recover as quickly as possible. Ask them about everything they are doing and if they can teach you how to better help your child.
- Unfortunately, as in every profession, there are medical personnel who are incompetent. Do not be afraid to request that certain people NOT work with you or your child. Most of our nurses were wonderful except for one. I had a strange feeling about her so I stuck right by Kellen when she was on duty. Luckily, we only had her one time.

- If possible, have someone stay with your child around the clock while he/she is in the hospital. If you are in the room with your child, you may be able to help them right away, as the nurses can be busy with other patients. You will also be able to prevent unnecessary medications or repeated tests on your child if you or someone is there to monitor this. I slept in a recliner right next to Kellen the whole time he was in the hospital because I couldn't sleep unless I was right by him. I also felt better about being there in case the nurses were busy and he needed something.

- Do not be afraid to speak your mind, but be friendly about it. Use "I" statements such as "I feel frustrated when…." You will not offend the medical staff this way, and will get your message across. You get further with sugar than you do with salt!

- Don't underestimate the value of the friendships that you can make with the staff at the hospital or doctor's office. By working together in a friendly manner, everyone wins!

- Review your child's medical chart. You will find a wealth of information in it and you can request to review the chart with the medical staff if necessary.

- Learn the medical language so that you can understand what the doctors and nurses are talking about.

- Always go with your gut feeling. If you feel uncomfortable about a procedure that must be done, it is acceptable to ask if there are other options available that might yield the same results.

Insurance Companies and HMO's

- Develop a working relationship with your insurance company or HMO. Keep detailed records (in your notebook) of whom you spoke to, what was said or promised, and what you said you would do in return.

- Prepare to do battle to get procedures paid for. Some insurance companies/HMO's won't pay until some procedures have been reviewed repeatedly. Be sure to contact the hospital in order to provide specific codes for certain procedures. *Insurance companies will pay if a specific code is used, and will not if the incorrect code is used.*

- Do not be too proud to ask for help if you cannot afford to pay your share of the procedures. You may be referred to the social work office for additional financial help. Many institutions will reduce the cost or eliminate your obligation to them, once they realize how extensive the medical issues are for your child.

You and your child

- Breastfeed your child if possible. Breast milk boosts the immune system and has many other health benefits for your baby, so this will be important after the operation. Many hospitals have "pumping rooms" that are already set up for mothers to have some privacy while pumping milk. Generally, there is an organized system at the hospital to freeze and store the breast milk for later use. It was exhausting, but am so glad that I pumped my milk for Kellen. I believe that the antibodies in the milk helped him to recover more quickly from the operation.

- Don't forget to appreciate the little things. Never forget to be amazed by your child's face. Cherish the time you spend with your child and be grateful that you are able to get your child the medical care he or she needs. This is not an option in many other parts of the world. Read a book, sing a song, and rock him or her for hours. Tell your older children that the baby is so lucky to have him/her for a big brother or sister. Treasure the time you have with your baby.

Preparing your older child for surgery or a stay in the hospital

- Start reading books like "Franklin Goes to the Hospital" (a good one and even goes into some detail on anesthesia), and "Clifford's Hospital Visit" (funny and makes the hospital not such a scary concept).

- Find a suitcase at the thrift store and spray paint it. Decorate it with the child's name stenciled on it and add your child's favorite pictures. You could include family pictures as well as pictures of the family pet. Make this the special "hospital suitcase" and let your child pick cd's and toys to put in it.

- Some hospitals have a "play therapist" who can work with your child on the pre-op day using a small operating room with bears for the doctors or patients, and letting them see what the doctors masks look like etc....this will help the child to be less fearful when going in for the operation.

Dealing with anxiety and fear when you have a sick child

- Having a critically ill child is extremely stressful. The fear and uncertainty can seem overwhelming at times. One thing I found helpful was to write everything down in a journal (which later turned out to be parts of this book). Writing out your feelings can be therapeutic, as well as informational. You may need to refer back to your journal at times.

- Be sure to BREATHE! While under stress, we forget to breathe properly. This can initiate panic attacks. Just taking some deep breaths will help immensely.

- Exercise—take a walk around the hospital if you are too afraid to leave your child. Being a former runner, I found running the hospital stairs to be a good way to let off excess steam. Exercise releases endorphins, which help to reduce the stress of having a sick child. I did eventually have to take anxiety medication because I started having panic attacks after Kellen's ordeal. My face and arms would go numb (at first I thought I was having a stroke), but once I learned the signs of the attacks, I was able to just breathe and get through them.

FURTHER TESTING AND HIRSCHSPRUNG'S DISEASE

Colon manometry

In some cases of Hirschsprung's Disease, it is necessary for the patient to undergo a colon manometry. A colon manometry will tell the doctor if the patient is having functional constipation or HD. During this test, the child is sedated for the placement of the catheter. The catheter is placed through the anus to the *cecum* (beginning of the large intestine). As the child awakes from sedation, the colon study begins. After about an hour, the child eats which initiates the gastrocolonic response (*peristalsis*). In a normal child and in children with functional constipation, the colon makes high amplitude propagating contractions (HAPCs). These contractions propel the colon contents toward the anus. In a patient with neuropathy in the colon, these contractions are absent. Through the biofeedback, the examiner can tell the child that the sensations are normal and that having a bowel movement will relieve his/her discomfort.

Anal manometry

After the child has been given a sedative, doctors place a balloon inside of the rectum. The balloon is then inflated with water at various points along the rectum (see Figure 48). In a normal person, the anal muscles (*sphincters*) will relax. This is a nerve reflex that occurs in most people. The internal anal sphincter is naturally in a state of constriction and relaxes in response to stretching of the rectum. This is called the anorectal inhibitory reflex (ARIR). If the sphincter muscle does not relax, HD could be the problem (see Figure 49).

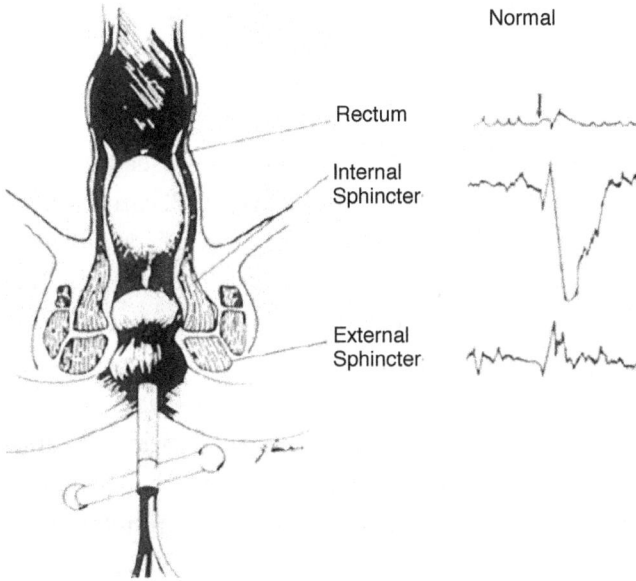

Figure 48. Manometer, anal balloon, and anal sphincter balloon are placed in the rectum. In a normal reaction, inflation of the rectal balloon causes a reflex relaxation of the internal anal sphincter muscles, and a contraction of the external anal sphincter muscles.

Image reprinted with permission from Wikimedia Commons, 2011.

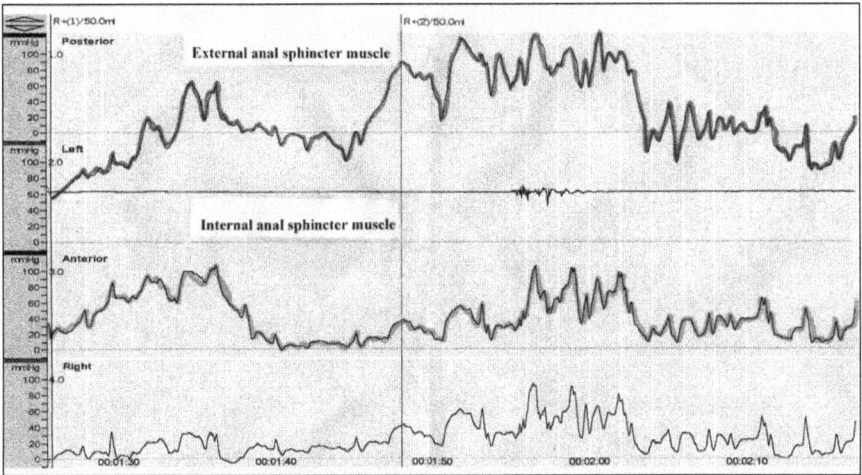

Figure 49. Anal manometry reading showing contractions of the internal anal sphincter and external anal sphincter muscles.

Anal manometry reading for Kellen Murphy.
Good Samaritan Hospital, Portland, Oregon. April 17, 2006.

STOMA CARE TIPS

By Monica Forte

Our son Tony has TCHD. He has an ileostomy (see figure 50) and will actually pull off his bag if he wants attention. Because Tony can sometimes have high ostomy outputs, we use a two-piece *urostomy bag* (bags used to collect urine after bladder surgery). Patients who have a stoma due to urinary or bladder problems will use these bags.

In our experience, the urostomy bags work the best. If the child doesn't pull the bag off, the bags will usually last 3-4 days. My husband and I always get compliments from Tony's doctors and nurses on how healthy his skin looks, especially around the *stoma* (a surgically-constructed opening, especially one in the abdominal wall that permits the passage of waste after a colostomy or ileostomy).

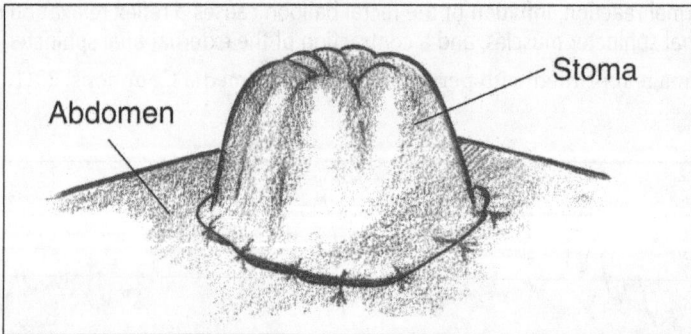

Figure 50. The word *stoma* comes from the Greek word meaning mouth or opening.

Image reprinted with permission from The National Institute of Diabetes and Digestive and Kidney Diseases, National Institute of Health, 2010.

Bag changing instructions

1. When taking off the bag, use an adhesive remover so as to not to irritate the skin.
2. Wipe off the area around the stoma using just a wet paper towel with **NO SOAP**. (The bar or lotion soap has oils it and can prevent the wafer from adhering to the skin).

3. Blot the skin with a dry paper towel and let it air dry. To prevent a mess with ostomy output, we use an **unscented** tampon. This works well because it absorbs the liquid and you can work around it. Make sure that the tampon is unscented because the perfumes in the scented ones can cause the skin to become irritated.

4. Sprinkle the stoma powder sparingly just around the base of the stoma. If there is any irritation, more of the powder can be applied.

5. Use the no sting barrier film lollipops and work around the stoma to the outer edge of where the bag ends. Fan dry so that there will be a good adhesion with the wafer.

6. Eakin Cohesive® Seals (http://www.eakin.co.uk) are a putty-like substance which can be molded around the stoma opening. The Eakin seal works wonderfully because it acts as a barrier for the skin around the stoma (https://www.edgepark.com), extends the life of the bag, and prevents skin irritations around the stoma. The seals come in four discs. Cut the disc like a pie in sections and use a small amount. Mold around the stoma.

7. The wafer comes with a precut hole in it. Place the hole over the stoma. Remove the backing and place around the Eakin seal, stoma, and skin. Press gently around the seal using the warmth of your fingers to mold to the skin.

8. The urostomy bag has a ring that snaps onto the wafer. Make sure the spout is closed and the snap is snapped (it locks). The spout works well because it allows for easy access while emptying the ostomy and it is more sanitary. The two-piece system is great because if your doctor needs to catheterize the stoma or perform a study, the bag can be removed but the wafer remains intact.

9. Finally, use *DuoDERM*® (a skin dressing used to protect skin while it heals) extra-thin to secure the wafer. It is almost like skin and you can cut it into strips. Place the strips around the wafer. This reinforces the bond between the wafer and the skin making it harder for babies and children to remove.

MICKEY BUTTON CARE TIPS

By Moncia Forte

Mickey button

In some cases of Hirschsprung's Disease it is necessary for the child to have a gastrostomy tube placed into the stomach during the newborn period. After about three weeks, the g-tube can be replaced with a mickey button. A Mic-Key® is a button that is placed in a surgical hole in the stomach. This button allows for venting of gas as well as feeding or hydrating a child when the child will not or cannot eat or drink. The mickey button (see Figure 51) is also useful for administering medications directly into the stomach.

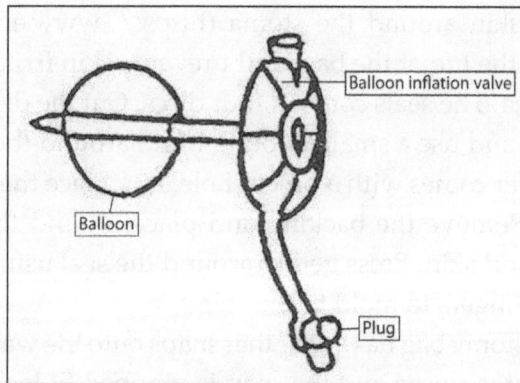

Figure 51. Mic-Key® button.
Image reprinted with permission from www.universityhospital.org

Changing the mickey button

1. Put on gloves.
2. Have a cup of sterile water and gauze handy.
3. While the mickey is in place, remove the flap that closes the mickey when not in use.

4. Insert the empty syringe into the hole of the mickey button and pull back gently. This will empty about 5 milliliters (same as a cc) of the water that was in the balloon.

5. Discard the water and rinse the syringe with water.

6. Put the syringe into the sterile cup of water drawing out about 5 ml (check with your doctor on this amount).

7. Before putting the mickey button into the stomach hole, insert the tip of the syringe into the hole of the mickey button and release the water slowly into the balloon. This will refill the balloon so that it can be checked for leaks.

8. Lubricate the end of the button to be inserted with preferred lubricant.

9. Repeat step 7 but this time put the mickey button into the hole in the stomach.

10. Close the flap

11. Wipe any excess water around the skin of the mickey

12. Check to see if the button can move with ease, as it cannot be too loose or too tight.

11. Be sure to always keep two extra mickey buttons on hand in case the original one dislodges. It is a good idea to have two on hand in case one has a leak in it. If the button comes out accidentally, follow the directions to replace it or go to the nearest emergency room to have it replaced. **It only takes about 2 hours for the hole to close, which would entail another surgery—so get there quickly.**

12. On a daily basis, clean the skin around the mickey with mild soap and water. If any redness appears around the site, apply some Neosporin onto the skin.

13. The leakage from the stomach acids can burn the skin around the button. In this case, an antacid like Maalox® can be applied. Let the antacid sit in a small container for about an hour. Pour off the watery liquid on top and apply the thick antacid onto the skin. A skin barrier like Aquaphor® can be used if the irritation is not relieved by the antacid.

14. Check the mickey button weekly in case it needs changing.

TOTAL PARENTERAL NUTRITION AND HIRSCHSPRUNG'S DISEASE

Total parenteral nutrition (TPN)

Total parenteral nutrition is the practice of feeding a person through an IV in order to bypass the gut. It is normally used following surgery, when feeding by mouth is not possible. The most common method of delivering TPN is with a medical infusion pump. The pump delivers a small amount of the *nutrient solution* (water, glucose, salts, amino acids, vitamins, and fats) continuously in order to keep the vein open. Insulin may be added to the infusion because blood sugar can increase with TPN (Wikipedia, 2007).

After surgery for HD, the gut must rest, so patients are put on TPN. In some cases of HD, the child will remain on TPN for an extended period of time. The most common complication of TPN use is bacterial infection. Bacterial infection is usually due to the increased infection risk from having an indwelling central venous catheter.

Line infections

Ninety percent of all catheter related blood stream infections are associated with central lines and only 10 percent with *peripheral lines* (venous lines) (Howard, 1996). The bacteria or fungus can move down the outside of the catheter or can become imbedded in the internal lining of the catheter causing infection. If infection is suspected, the blood will be cultured to determine what kind of bacteria is to blame.

TPN LINE CARE TIPS
By Monica Forte

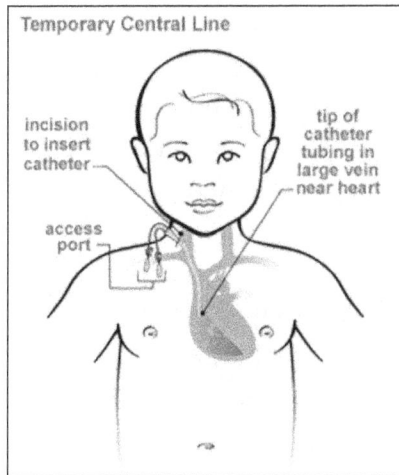

Figure 52. Position of TPN/central line.
Image reprinted with permission from Wikimedia Commons, 2011.

Preventing central line infections

Line infections are common with *TPN* (Total Parenteral Nutrition) (see Figure 52). It is rare that a patient on TPN will go without having some sort of infection. Because the TPN solution used is mostly made of sugar, the bacteria on our skin or in the air will cling to the sugar. This is why sterilization is the key to keeping the patient healthy. It is also important that whomever is accessing the line (parents or RN) be properly trained in line care. Multiple unnecessary line infections can occur if proper precautions are not made. It is also a good idea to have the same person access the line as exposure to different types of bacteria is decreased.

Infection can also occur during changing of the dressing. The steps needed for dressing changes vary from hospital to hospital but should be done in a sterile environment. When the child on TPN is at home, a changing station can be set up in the child's' bedroom preferably away from the other children in the family.

Organizing TPN supplies

All necessary supplies can be kept in clear office supply bins. The three tier bins are useful because they are stackable and can hold more supplies while taking up less space. A tackle box can be purchased to hold the line supplies. Having extra ostomy supplies available for unexpected midnight trips to the hospital is also helpful. Clear office supply bins can be used to organize the TPN supplies. Each bin can be labeled in the following manner: Heparin flushes, Saline flushes, Alcohol swabs, etc.

Materials needed for changing the dressing

Anyone helping or accessing the line must wash, sanitize and glove hands as well as wear a mask. Be sure to look for drainage or redness around the site during changing. This could be a sign of a line infection. It is also important to check the blood return in the line to be sure no clots have formed and a new line is not needed.

The following items are necessary when changing the dressing:
- Three alcohol swab sticks (large Q-tips)
- Three Providone-iodine (for disinfecting) swab sticks
- Three alcohol swab sticks (for disinfecting)
- One mini-island dressing
- Two mini-island *tegaderms* (a thin sterile dressing that keeps germs away from the skin, yet lets the skin breathe)
- One large tegaderm
- One chlorprep (a one-step system used to clean the site) dressing kit

Guidelines for changing the dressing

1. Be sure everyone involved is gloved and masked.
2. Open the chlorprep dressing kit and the swab stick packages.

3. While one person holds the child, use adhesive remover to help peel away the tegaderm. Be sure not to get any on the insertion site.

4. The person doing the dressing change can remove his/her gloves and put on the sterile gloves. While being careful not to touch the wrapper, the person holding the child can hand the package of alcohol swab sticks to the person changing the dressing.

5. Gently remove the swab stick and put the swab stick on the insertion site. Move in a circle away from the site to the outer edge being sure not to reuse the swab stick or go back in the circle with the same stick.

6. Take the next alcohol stick and repeat step five.

7. Using the iodine swab stick, repeat step five, each time cleaning the line all of the way down. Repeat this process three times. Be sure to let the line AIR DRY as blowing or waving near the insertion site can force unwanted bacteria onto the line.

8. Take the next set of three alcohol swab sticks and repeat the previous steps. This time, wipe off any of the remaining iodine.

9. Make a safety loop with the line being careful not to have the line on the insertion site. Put mini island cloth dressing on facing east and west (horizontally).

10. Take two mini tegaderms and cover the edges in a vertical fashion (back to back). Then take a large tegaderm and place it horizontally over the entire dressing.

11. Take two more mini tegaderms and tape the catheter to the child. This will prevent pulling on the line during the infusion.

12. To minimize infection during the infusion, anyone around the child should be sanitized, masked and gloved. Always use a new alcohol swab between breaking the line and infusing the saline. Wipe the end of the catheter with a new swab and then again wipe the catheter tip after infusing the heparin.

The parents can also be trained in preparing the bag of TPN that contains the drugs *ranitidine* (reduces stomach acid production) and *heparin* (stops blood from clotting). Generally, the infusion is done with a syringe so it is necessary to put a sharp container in the child's room away from the other children in the family.

Having a parent stay in the hospital with the child is very important. The parent can then assist the nurses during the whole process, as it is impossible for medical staff to know each parents preferences. It is also imperative that anyone working with the child including medical staff is gloved and masked.

Signs of a line infection

During an onset of a line infection, the child may vomit and have the shakes *(rigors)*. A sharp spike in temperature is also a sign that a trip to the hospital is imminent. It is extremely important to have a standing order written by the doctor at the hospital for children who are frequently admitted. This way, the ER can be bypassed the child can be directly admitted into the pediatric unit. Generally, the doctors will start the child on antibiotics as a precaution until the cultures come back. This allows the doctors to see what type of bacteria is involved permitting them to use the appropriate antibiotics.

An *npo* (nothing by mouth) order and an IV help the child to get rehydrated. Calling the pediatric surgeons while on the way to the hospital gives the doctors and nurses time to prepare for the ill child. In some cases, the child may need a blood transfusion due to the amount of blood needed for the labs.

This process seems long at first, but after awhile, it goes quickly. When the parents aren't home, it is important to have the nurses caring for the child watch the process so that they know how to do it properly. There are health care organizations that will come and change the dressing once a week (Horizon Health Care in our case).

SYNDROMES ASSOCIATED WITH HIRSCHSPRUNG'S DISEASE

In 70% of cases, Hirschsprung's Disease occurs as an isolated trait. Twelve percent of HD patients have an associated abnormality with Hirschsprung's Disease and the final 18% of patients have associated chromosomal abnormalities. The most frequent of these anomalies is Trisomy 21, better known as Down syndrome. Down syndrome occurs in about 2-10% of HD cases (Ameil, Lyonnet, 2001). Along with a rare form of cancer called neuroblastoma, there are other syndromes and isolated anomalies associated with Hirschsprung's Disease.

Down syndrome

In 1866, a physician named Langdon Down published an essay in England describing a set of children with common features in an asylum for children with mental retardation. Down was the superintendent of the asylum and noticed that these children were different from the others. Some physical features he noticed were low muscle tone, flattish facial features, an upward eye slant, a protruding tongue, and a single crease across the palm of the hand. People with Down syndrome have an increased chance of infection, childhood leukemia, heart defects and respiratory problems. He first called the children "mongoloids," but the term was dropped in the early 1960s after protest from Asian genetic researchers.

In 1959, Jerome Lejeune and Patricia Jacobs determined that the cause of Down syndrome lies on Chromosome 21. Human cells normally have 46 chromosomes, which are arranged in 23 pairs. Of these 23, 22 (the *autosomal* chromosomes) are alike in males and females; the 23rd pair is comprised of the sex chromosomes (X & Y). Each member of a pair of chromosomes carries the same information, meaning that the same genes are in the same spots on the chromosome. Variations of that gene or "alleles" may be present. For example, the genetic information for eye color is a "gene" but the variations for blue, brown or green are the "alleles."

A normal set of chromosomes has 22 evenly paired chromosomes along with the sex chromosomes, equaling 23 pairs. The XX means that a person is a female and an XY means that the person is a male. Children with Down syndrome have three of the 21st chromosome instead of only two (see Figure 53). A karotype is a test in which blood samples are checked for the number and type of chromosomes.

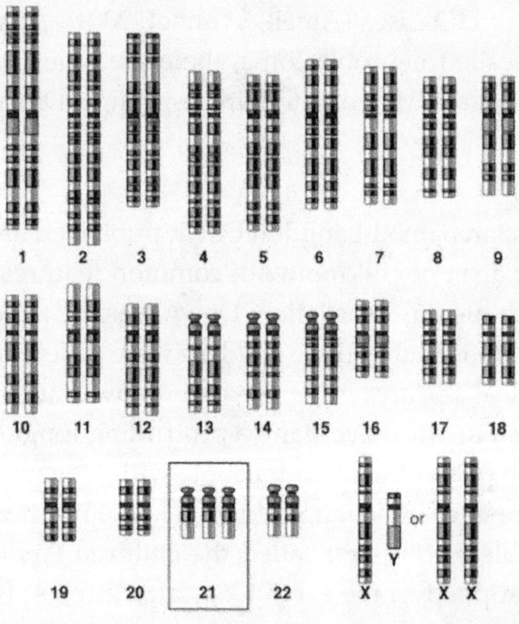

Figure 53. A genetic mapping of Trisomy 21 (Down syndrome).
Image courtesy of the National Human Genome Research Institute, www.genome.gov, 2010.

During cell division, many errors can occur. If a sperm or an egg cell has an abnormal number of chromosomes and they merge with a normal mate, the resulting fertilized egg will have an abnormal number of chromosomes. This accident is called "nondisjunction." In Down syndrome (DS), 95% of cases are caused by this event (Leshin, 2003). For this to occur, either the egg or sperm cell would have to have had two 21st chromosomes instead of one *(nondisjunction)*. It has been shown recently through research that around 90% of these cases are caused by an abnormal egg cell. Maternal age plays a key role in the nondisjunction error and more is being researched on this topic.

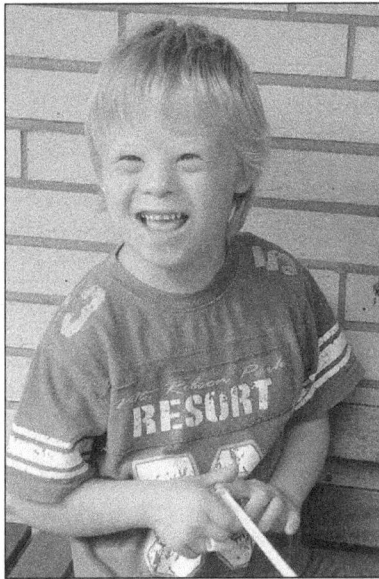

Figure 54. Little boy with Down syndrome.
Image reprinted with permission from Wikimedia Commons, 2010.

Over expression of genes occurs when there is an extra chromosome. This leads to increased production of certain materials that the body needs. There are many unique features associated with Down syndrome. A wide range of mental retardation and developmental delay is noted in Down syndrome children. Other complications Down babies can have are heart problems, epilepsy, hypothyroidism, celiac disease and Hirschsprung's Disease.

Hirschsprung's Disease in a constipated infant with Down syndrome was first noted in Cuba by Vacher, Garcia, and Palacio (1956). Fewer than three percent of Down syndrome children have HD, and around two to 10% of those with Hirschsprung's Disease have Down syndrome (Albertus, 2006). It is believed that there is at least one gene on chromosome 21, which is implicated in Hirschsprung's Disease when present in two defective copies. HD can also be caused by genes on other chromosomes and inherited in different ways. According to Julie Albertus, genetics counselor at Johns Hopkins University, studying syndromic forms of HD, like DS, can help researchers find new genes involved in causing Hirschsprung's Disease.

Shah-Waardenburg syndrome

Shah-Waardenburg syndrome (WS4) is a condition characterized by deafness and *partial albinism* (the absence of pigmentation), including a white forelock and eyelashes, very pale blue eyes or two different colored eyes, areas of skin without pigment, and Hirschsprung's Disease (see Figure 55). Mutations on the SOX10, EDNRB and EDN3 genes have been recently noted (Ameil & Lionnet, 2001). Shah-Waardenburg syndrome seems to also be autosomal dominant but may skip some family members and look different in other family members. In the Mennonite population, WS4 may be autosomal recessive, meaning that both parents must pass the gene onto their offspring for the syndrome to develop (Albertus, 2006).

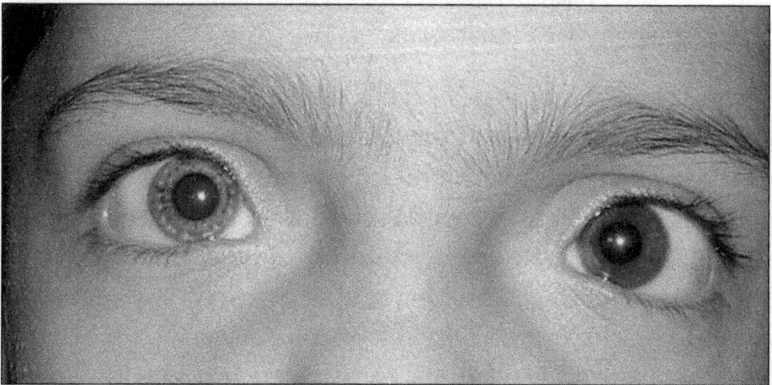

Figure 55. Hetero-chromia (two different colored eyes).
Image reprinted with permission from Wikimedia Commons, 2010.

Ondine's curse

Ondine was a beautiful and immortal water nymph in German mythology. The only threat to her eternal happiness was that if she fells in love with a mortal and bore his child, she would lose her gift of everlasting life.

Ondine fell in love with a handsome knight named Sir Lawrence and they were married. Sir Lawrence, during their vows, said, "My every waking breath shall be my pledge of love and faithfulness to you." One year later, their son was born and from that moment on, Ondine began to age. As her physical attractiveness faded, Lawrence lost interest in his wife.

One afternoon, Ondine was walking near the stables when she heard her husband snoring. When she entered the stable, she saw Sir Lawrence lying in the arms of another woman. Ondine kicked her husband awake, pointed her finger at him, and cursed him saying, "You swore faithfulness to me with every waking breath, and I accepted your oath. So be it. As long as you are awake, you shall have your breath, but should you ever fall asleep, then that breath will be taken from you and you will die!" (Wikipedia Encyclopedia, 2005).

Identified about 30 years ago, central alveolar hypoventilation syndrome (CCHS), Ondine's curse, is a respiratory disorder that is fatal if left untreated (Amiel & Lionnet, 2001). People affected with Ondine's curse are unable to breathe without conscious intervention; if they fall asleep, they will die. The central nervous system fails to control breathing while the person is asleep; however, people with Ondine's curse can survive if they are kept alive with a ventilator at night. CCHS patients often have other symptoms, such as neural crest cell derived tumors. The gene responsible for CCHS is called PHOX2B. If the people affected by it have children, their children will have a 50% chance of also being affected.

The combination of Hirschsprung's Disease and CCHS is called Haddad syndrome (MIM 209880). HD is noted in around 14-20% of CCHS patients (Amiel & Lyonnet, 2005). The majority of cases of CCHS are caused by mutations in PHOX2B; however, mutations in other genes, such as RET, EDN3 and GDNF genes, have been noted in patients with or without a PHOX2B mutation. Whether they contribute to the disease is not known. Some patients with CCHS have down slanting eyes, a small nose, a triangular-shaped mouth, and ears that are low-set and backwards rotated. These characteristics, however, are not essential in making a diagnosis for Haddad syndrome.

Mowat-Wilson syndrome

It has been only in the last few years that Mowat-Wilson syndrome has been defined. It is associated with many malformations, mainly in the face, and causes mental retardation. Previously called Hirschsprung-mental retardation syndrome, other features include delayed motor development, epilepsy, small head *(microcephaly)*, cleft palate, sparse scalp hair, heart defects, short stature, and learning disabilities. Other characteristics of this syndrome are Hirschsprung's Disease, rotated ears, respiratory distress, a v-shaped mouth, a broad nose bridge, and feeding difficulties (see Figure 56).

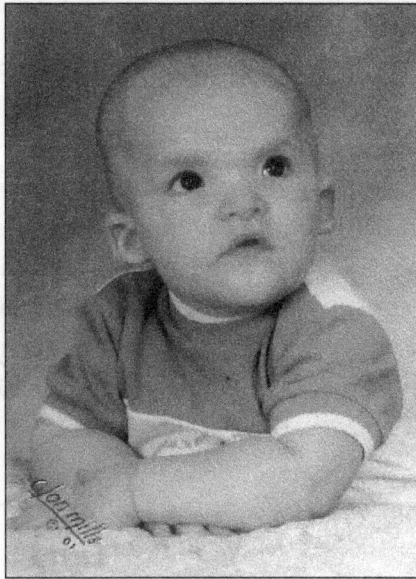

Figure 56. A baby with Mowat-Wilson syndrome.
Image reprinted with permission from "Jablonski's syndromes database," 2005.
www.mowatwilson.org

Goldberg-Shprintzen syndrome (GSS)

Goldberg-Shprintzen syndrome is a rare disorder in which there are multiple abnormalities at birth. In this syndrome, there is a combination of Hirschsprung's Disease, cleft palate, decreased muscle tone, a small head, and mental retardation. Dysmorphic facial features like a prominent nose and broad nose bridge, sparse hair, and large ears are a few of the features that may be present (see Figure 57). Internally, a person with GSS can have heart defects and brain atrophy. An irregular density of white matter on the brain may suggest a defect in neuronal migration to this area (Amiel & Lyonnet, 2001).

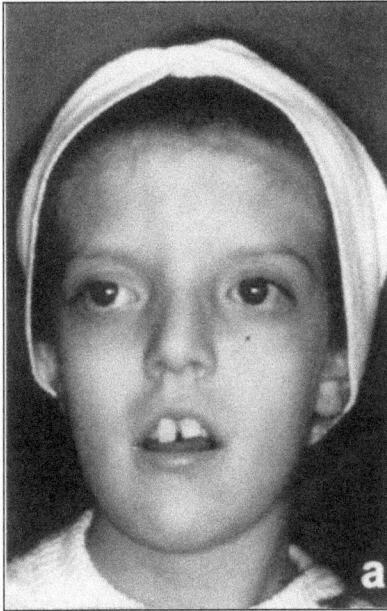

Figure 57. A young girl with Goldberg-Shprintzen syndrome (GSS).

Image reprinted with permission from *The Cleft Palate-Craniofacial Journal*. 2007.
http://cpcj.allenpress.com

Cartilage-hair hypoplasia syndrome (CHH)

First described in the Old Order Amish community in 1965, CHH is a disorder that causes short limb dwarfism, thin sparse and blond hair, and immunity problems (see Figure 58). Hirschsprung's Disease occurs in about 10% of these cases (Amiel & Lyonnet, 2001). CHH patients are extremely susceptible to the chicken pox virus. Many CHH patients are also anemic and some cases are so severe, that they can die of it.

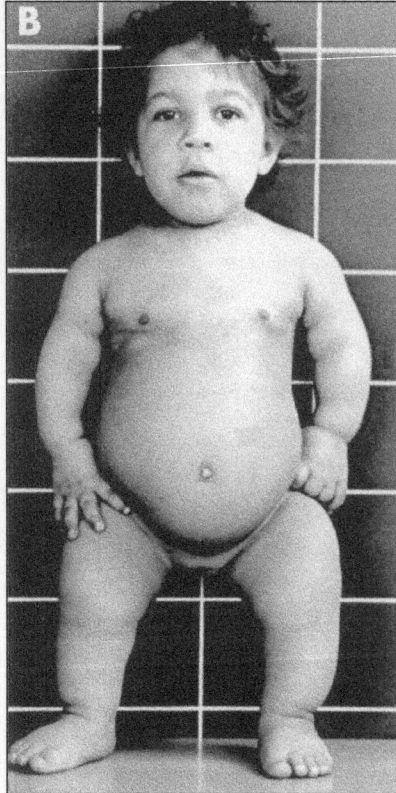

Figure 58. A young child with CHH.
Image reprinted with permission from the Geneva Foundation for Medical Education & Research, 2010.

Bardet-Biedl syndrome (BBS)

Bardet-Biedl syndrome is a complex disorder affecting many parts of the body. This syndrome is usually diagnosed in childhood when visual problems become apparent. The *retina* (thin membrane at the back of the eyeball) begins to degenerate causing night blindness and a loss of *peripheral vision* (tunnel vision). People with BBS also have vision loss during childhood or adolescence. The symptoms are very similar to retinitis pigmentosa (RP) and can lead to severe visual impairment by early adulthood.

Polydactyly (extra fingers and/or toes) and obesity are other characteristics of Bardet-Biedl syndrome. This syndrome can be suspected when a child is born with polydactyly. Webbing between the fingers and toes is also common with this syndrome. Individuals can have short, broad feet and are sometimes shorter than average (Foundation Fighting Blindness, 2007).

Around half of all people with BBS have developmental disabilities ranging from mild impairment to mental retardation. According to geneticist Julie Albertus, a majority of individuals have significant learning difficulties, but only a minority have severe impairment on IQ testing. Individuals with BBS can also have kidney disease and smaller than average genitalia. Females with Bardet-Biedl syndrome can have irregular menstrual cycles. Hirschsprung's Disease has been reported in several BBS cases (Amiel & Lyonnet, 2001).

Smith-Lemli-Opitz syndrome (SLOS)

SLOS is a genetic disorder that affects the development of children both before and after birth. This syndrome was first explained in 1964 by geneticists Smith, Lemli, and Opitz. In 1993, scientists discovered that children with SLOS are unable to utilize cholesterol because they are lacking the enzyme needed to break it down.

Smith Lemli-Opitz syndrome is associated with multiple abnormalities (see Figure 59). Some of the characteristics of SLOS are; slow growth, small head, moderate to severe mental retardation, Hirschsprung's Disease, and other malformations. Common malformations include; low-set ears, cleft palate, heart defects, cataracts, *ptosis* (drooping eyelids), *pyloric stenosis* (narrowing of the lower part of the stomach), small chin, short thumbs, underdeveloped external genitalia in males, *hypospadias* (abnormally placed urinary opening) in males, undescended testicles, polydactyly, and *syndactyly* (webbing) of the toes (NCBI Bookshelf, 2009).

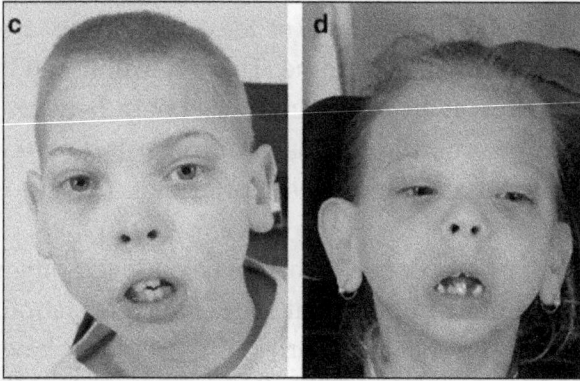

Figure 59. Facial characteristics of Smith-Lemli-Opitz syndrome.
Image reprinted with permission from www.nature.com, 2009.

ISOLATED ANOMALIES
AND HIRSCHSPRUNG'S DISEASE

In addition to the above syndromes, many isolated anomalies (irregularities) have been described in cases of HD. In 5% of Hirschsprung's cases, heart defects are found. Limb abnormalities like polydactyly can also exist as well as other gastrointestinal malformations. "Other health problems can be a sign that there is an underlying syndrome causing HD and examination by a geneticist is important in these cases" (Albertus, 2006).

Abnormal facial features are frequently found by trained *dysmorphologists* (someone who studies abnormal body features). It is also important to have skeletal x-rays and cardiac and urogenital echographic surveys done in patients with HD. These procedures can rule out other problems Hirschsprung's patients can have and in some cases may lead to identification of a syndrome (Amiel & Lyonnet, 2005).

Neuroblastoma

Neuroblastoma is a form of cancer that occurs in infants and young children. It is a malignant tumor formed of embryonic ganglion cells. It is rarely found in children older than 10 years of age. Hirschsprung's Disease, Ondine's curse (CCHS) and neuroblastoma are all *neurocristopathies* (disease caused by a developmental anomaly of the neural crest). Some children affected by CCHS also have some form of neuroblastoma and 16-20% have HD or Haddad syndrome (CCHS & HD together).

Two thirds of neuroblastomas start in the abdomen and one-third start in the adrenal glands, located on top of the kidneys. The remaining neuroblastomas begin in the chest, neck, or pelvis. Unfortunately, screening tests for this kind of cancer have proven unsuccessful (CRI, 2005).

Neuroblastoma can cause strange changes in children's bodies due to a release of hormones. Some symptoms of neuroblastoma are diarrhea, strange eye movements, and spastic muscles, high blood pressure, rapid heartbeat, sweating, and reddening of the skin. Successful treatment depends on the type of neuroblastoma and the stage at which it is diagnosed.

Multiple endocrine neoplasia type two (MEN 2)

Multiple endocrine neoplasia type two is a hereditary form of thyroid cancer. Also known as Sipple syndrome, it is named for the person who discovered it in 1961 (Carney, 2005). There are two types of this cancer: MEN 2A and MEN 2B. A person with MEN 2A can have adrenal pheochromocytomas, parathyroid tumors, and cancer of the thyroid gland. MEN 2A is an autosomal dominant condition, meaning that children of an affected individual are at a 50% risk to inherit the disease. MEN 2A is caused by activating mutations in the RET gene, whereas HD is caused by a loss of function mutation in the RET gene. Most families have either MEN 2A or HD, not both however; a few individuals have been described with both conditions (Albertus, 2006).

Adrenal pheochromocytomas are tumors of the adrenal gland. The adrenal glands are located on the top of each kidney and produce the hormone adrenaline. Adrenaline helps to maintain blood pressure and allows the body to cope with stressful situations. Some symptoms of pheochromocytomas are severe headaches, sweating, heart palpitations, anxiety, tremors, abdominal pain, nausea, weight loss, and heat intolerance.

BOWEL MANAGEMENT
AND HIRSCHSPRUNG'S DISEASE

Fecal incontinence can have various negative implications for the children involved. Multi-disciplinary behavioral treatments have been developed that have greatly helped children with chronic defecation problems after HD surgery. These treatments teach the child about bowel self-control, adequate straining techniques, and extinction of fear of going to the bathroom.

These treatments are carried out by a child psychologist, a pediatric physiotherapist, and a pediatric surgeon (Van Kuyk, Brugman, Wissink, Severijnen, Festen, and Bleijenberg, 2000). Dr. Marc Levitt, and Dr. Alberto Pena have developed a Bowel Management Program at The Colorectal Center for Children in Cincinnati, Ohio. They have treated over 500 patients and have had a 95% success rate. (Levitt & Pena, 2007).

The Bowel Management Program designed by Dr. Levitt and Dr. Pena teaches the patient or his/her parents how to do an enema to keep the colon clean daily. This allows the child to keep his/her underwear clean for a 24-hour period. Each day, the patient is seen and an x-ray is taken of the abdomen. This allows the doctors to determine how much stool is left in the colon so that adjustments to the individualized program can be made.

When the child grows old enough to do the enemas on his/her own, a continent appendicostomy (also known as the Malone or ACE procedure) can be performed if necessary. A small opening in the belly button is constructed through which the patient can pass a small catheter into the colon (see Figure 60). The child can then administer the enemas themselves while sitting on the toilet, thus allowing for more independence (Levitt & Pena, 2005).

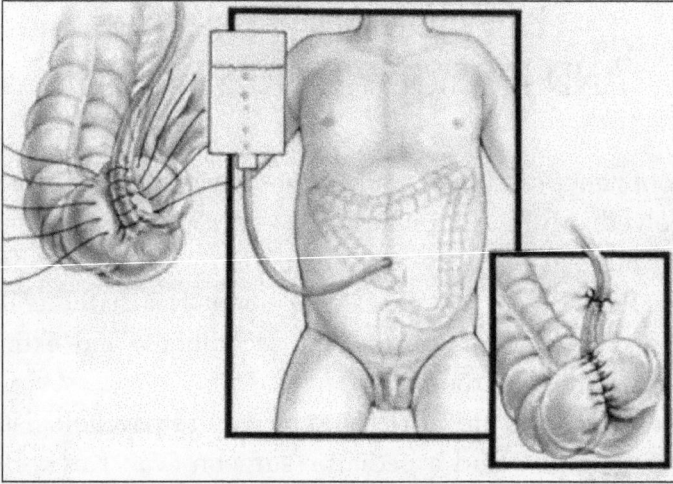

Figure 60. In a Malone appendicostomy, the appendix is used to attach a permanent catheter to the colon making this procedure quicker and easier for the patient.

Image reprinted with permission from Levitt, Soffer, and Pena, (2010).

Parents of children who suffer from diarrhea or loose stool are given a list of constipating foods to provide for their child. Foods that promote loose stools are avoided and the child is put on a rigid diet. Parents are encouraged to learn which foods constipate their child and which foods cause diarrhea. The treatment starts with enemas, a very strict diet, and Immodium® (an anti-diarrhea medication). Most children respond to this program within 24 hours and experience a new sense of confidence based on improved quality of life (Levitt & Pena, 2005).

HELPFUL WEBSITES

- ayearinthelifeofhirschsprungs.blogspot.com by Stella Taylor
- Hirschsprungshelp@yahoo.com
  (the group I started to help parents)
- Facebook site on Hirschsprung's Disease. Go to "Hirschsprung's Disease Help Book" to get weekly facts on HD as well as links to other HD sites.
- American Pediatric Surgical Association website: http://www.eapsa.org
- Baseline of Health Foundation (probiotics) website: http://www.jonbarron.org
- Cincinnati Children's Hospital, Colorectal Center website (Dr. Mark Levitt): http://www.cincinnatichildrens.org/health/info/abdomen/diagnose/hirschsprung.htm
- Institute of Child Health website: http://www.ich.ucl.ac.uk
- International Foundation for Functional Gastrointestinal Disorders website: www.iffgd.org
- International Pediatric Endosurgery Group website: http://www.ipeg.org
- Johns Hopkins University, Institute of Genetic Medicine, educational & study website (contact Courtney Nichols): cnichols@jhmi.edu
- Mayo Clinic (constipation/diaper rash) website: http://www.mayoclinic.com
- National Digestive Diseases Information Clearinghouse, NIDDK, and NIH website: http://digestive.niddk.nih.gov
- National Organization for Rare Disorders (NORD) website: http://www.rarediseases.org
- Pull-thru Network website: http://www.pullthrough.org

REFERENCES

A brain in the gut? (n.d.). Retrieved November 11, 2005, from
http://whyfiles.org

*A heterozygous endothelin 3 mutation in Waardenburg-Hirschsprung
disease.* (2001). Retrieved September 15, 2005, from
http://jmg.bmjjournals.com

About Kids, International Foundation For Gastrointestinal
Disorders. 2005 (April, 23rd). "What is Hirschsprung's disease."
http://www.aboutkidsgi.org

Action Medical Research. (2005). Brilliant boost for bowel research.
Retrieved June 7, 2005 from http://www.action.org.uk

Albertus, J., Genetics Coordinator. Johns Hopkins University Institute
of Genetic Medicine. hirschsprung@igm.jhmi.edu

American Pediatric Surgical Association. (2004).
Hirschsprung's disease. Retrieved May 6, from
http://www.epasa.org/parents/hirschsprungs3.htm

American Pediatric Surgical Association (2004). For Parents:
Hirschsprung's disease. Retrieved May 6, 2005, from
http://www.eapsa.org

Amiel, J., Lyonnet, S. (n.d.) *Hirschsprung's disease, associated
syndromes, and genetics: a review.* Retrieved August 10, 2005, from
http://jmg.bmjjournals.com

Arhan, P., Devroede, G., Danis, K., Dornic, C., Faverdin, B., Persoz, B.
(1978). Viscoelastic properties of the rectal wall in Hirschsprung's
disease. *The Journal of Clinical Investigation, 62,* 82-87.

Arnold, A., (n.d.) *The RET proto-oncogene and the MEN 2A syndrome -
clinical use of a genetic marker of disease.* Retrieved November 19,
2005, from http://www.bamc.amedd.army.mil

Aslam A., Spicer, R., Corfield, A., (1981). Enterocolitis associated with
Hirschsprung's disease. *Journal of Pediatric Surgery, 16,* 664.

Baseline of Health Foundation (1999). Intestinal health and digestive disorders. The probiotic miracle. Retrieved April 4, 2008, from www.jonbarron.org

Bill, J., & Chapman, N. (1962). The enterocolitis of Hirschsprung's disease: its natural history and treatment. *American Journal of Surgery, 103,* 70.

Cancer Reference Information. (2005). How Is neuroblastoma diagnosed? Retrieved October 21, from http://www.cancer.org

Cancer Reference Information. (2005). What is neuroblastoma? Retrieved October 21, 2005. http://www.cancer.org

Caniero, P., Brereton, R., Drake, D., Kiely, E., Spitz, L., and Turnock, R. (1992). Enterocolitis in Hirschsprung's disease. Evaluation of mortality and long-term function in 260 cases. *Archives of Surgery, 127,* 934.

Carney, J. (2005). Familial multiple endocrine neoplasia. *American Journal of Surgery, 2,* 254-74.

Cato-Smith, A., Coffey, C., Nolan T., Hutson, J. (1995). Fecal incontinence after the surgical treatment of Hirschsprung's disease. *Journal of Pediatric Gastroenterology & Nutrition, 127,* 954-957.

Children's Medical Encyclopedia. What is Hirschsprung's disease? (n.d.). Retrieved from http://www.childrenscentralcal.org

Cimarra, P., Nurko, S., Barksdale, El, Fishman S., Di Lorenzo, C. (2003). Internal anal sphincter achalasia in children: clinical characteristics and treatment with Clostridium botulinum toxin. *Journal of Pediatric Gastroenterology and Nutrition, 37,* 315-319.

Daigo, Y., Takayam, I., Ponder, B., Caldas, C., Ward, S., Sanders, K., Fujino, M. (2002). *Differential gene expression in the murine gastric fundus lacking interstitial cells of Cajal.* Retrieved November 14, 2005, from http://www.biomedcentral.com

Definition of Ondine's curse. (n.d.) Retrieved November 18, 2005, from http://www.medterms.com

De Caluwe, D., Yoneda A., Akl, U., Puri, P. (2001). Internal anal sphincter achalasia:

outcome after internal sphincter myectomy. *Journal of Pediatric Surgery, 36*, 736-738.

Dharmananda, S. Ph.D., (2009). Safety Issues Affecting Herbs: How Long can Stimulant Laxatives be Used? Institute for Traditional Medicine, Portland, Or.

Di Lorenzo, C., Solzi, G., Flores, A., Schwankovsky, L., Hyman, P. (2000). Colonic motility after surgery for Hirschsprung's Disease. *American Journal of Gastroenterology, 95*,1759-1764.

DNA, chromosomes and genes. (n.d.). Retrieved November 23, 2005, from http://www.ncc.gmu.edu

Donat, E. MD. 2005, (April, 22nd). "Hirschsprung's Disease." Retrieved March 28, 2006, from http://www.uottawa.ca/academic/med/cellmed/hirc.html

Dourmishev, A., MD, (2005). *Down Syndrome.* Retrieved November 21, 2005, from the Department of Dermatology and Venereology, Medical University, Sofia, Bulgaria: from http://www.emedicine.com

Down syndrome and Hirschsprung Disease. (n.d.) Retrieved November 19, 2005, from http://www.altonweb.com

Down Syndrome. (n.d.) Retrieved November 21, 2005, from http://www.encyclopedia.com

Drug Digest. (n.d.). Retrieved April 3, 2007, from http://www.drugdigest.org

Edery, P., Pelet, A., Mulligan, L., Abel, L., Attie, T., Dow, E., et al. (1994). Long segment and short segment familial Hirschsprung's: variable clinical expression at the RET locus. *Journal of Medical Genetics, 31*, 602-606.

Elhalaby, E., Teitelbaum, D., Coran, A., Heidelberger, K. (1995). Enterocolitis associated with Hirschsprung's disease: a clinical histopathological correlative study. *Journal of Pediatric Surgery, 30*, 1023.

Encopreis (2005). About your diagnosis. Retrieved June, 7, 2005, from http://www.lakeside.ca/Patient_Info/encopresis.htm

Encyclopedia of Medicine. Dehydration (n.d.) Retrieved March 30, 2007, from http://www.enotes.com

Fortuna, R., Weber, T., Tracy, T., Silen, M., Cradock, T. (1996). Critical analysis of operative treatment of Hirschsprung's disease. *Archives of Surgery, 131,* 520.

Fox, I. (1987). *Human Physiology, second edition.* Dubuque: WC Brown Publishers

Gariepy, C., Cass, D., Yanagisawa, M. (1996). Null mutation of endothelin receptor type B gene in spotting lethal rats causes aganglionic megacolon and white coat color. *Proc. Natl. Acad. Sci. USA, 93,* 867-872.

Gastroenteritis. (n.d.). Retrieved February 22, 2007, from http://www.answers.com

Gastrografin. (n.d.) Retrieved August, 14, 2007, from http://www.drugs.com

Gene secret of "mythical curse." (n.d.) Retrieved November 18, 2005, from http://news.bbc.co.uk

Genetics FAQ. (n.d.). Retrieved November 20, 2005, from http://www.genome.gov

Gershon, M. (1999). *The enteric nervous system: a second brain.* Retrieved November 11, 2005, from Columbia University: http://www.hosppract.com

Goldberg-Shprintzen megacolon syndrome. (n.d.). Retrieved November 20, 2005, from http://www.ncbi.nlm.nih.gov

Gura, K., Duggan C., Collier, S., Jennings, R., Folman, J., et al. (2006). Reversal of parenteral nutrition – associated liver disease in two infants with short bowel syndrome using parenteral fish oil: implications for future management. *Pediatrics, 118,* 197-201.

Hilton-Kamm, D. (2010). *Concerning Interactions with Doctors, Nurses and Medical Staff.* Retrieved January 2nd, 2011, from http://www.congenitalheartdefects.com/advice.html

Hamid, Syed, A., Di Lorenzo, C., Reddy, S., Narashimha., Flores, A., et al. (1998). Bisacodyl and high-amplitude-propagating colonic contractions in children. *Journal of Pediatric Gastroenterology & Nutrition, 27,* 398-402.

Harjai, M. (2000). Hirschsprung's disease: revisited. Retrieved January, 15, from http://www.surgical-tutor.org.uk/system/hnep/hirschsprungs.htm

Hirschsprung, H. (1888). Constipation in the newborn as a result of dilation and hypertrophy of the colon. *Springer, 24,* 408-410.

Hirschsprung, H. (n.d.). His life and medical career. Retrieved November 4, 2005, from Whonamedit.com

Hirschsprung's disease. (n.d.). Retrieved November 20, 2005, from http://www.humpath.com

Hirschsprung's disease - Mowat-Wilson syndrome. (n.d.) Retrieved November 20, 2005, from http://www.orpha.net

Hirschsprung's disease. (n.d.). Retrieved August 14, 2005, from University of Michigan-Pediatric Surgery: http://pediatric.um-surgery.org

Hofstra, R. (1999). *A consanguineous family with Hirschsprung disease, microcephaly, and mental retardation (Goldberg-Shprintzen syndrome).* Retrieved November 20, 2005, from http://jmg.bmjjournals.com

Huffnagle, G. (2006). Probiotics can be a key to good health. Retrieved May 20, 2008, from University of Michigan Health Systems, http://nutrition.about.com

Hyman, P. (2005). Defecation disorders after surgery for Hirschsprung's disease. *Journal of Pediatric Gastroenterology and Nutrition, 41,* S62-S63.

Hyperosmotic Laxatives, Oral. (n.d.). Retrieved April 3, 2007, from http://www.fairview.org

Hyperthyroidism. (n.d.) Retrieved November 19, 2005, from_ http://www.endocrineweb.com

Ikeda, K., Goto, S. (1986). Total colonic aganglionosis with or without small bowel involvement: an analysis of 137 patients. *Journal of Pediatric Surgery, 21,* 319-322.

Institute fur Humangenetik - *Mowat-Wilson syndrome.* (n.d.). Retrieved November 20, 2005, from http://www.hugenet

Institute of Child Health. (2005). Hirschsprung's Disease. Retrieved September 18, 2005, from http://www.ich.ucl.ac.uk

International Pediatric Endosurgery Group. (2004). Guidelines for surgical treatment of Hirschsprung's disease. Retrieved April 27, 2005, from http://www.ipeg.org

Irons, M., (1998). Smith-Lemli-Opitz syndrome. Retrieved June 10, 2009, from NCBI Bookshelf. http://www.ncbi.hlm.nih.gov.

Kaymakcioglu, N., Yagci, G., Can, M., Demiriz, M., Peker, Y., Akdeniz, A. (2005). Role of anorectal myectomy in the treatment of short segment Hirschsprung's disease in young adults. *Journal of International Surgery, 90*, 109-112.

Khaleghnejad-Tabari, A., Moslemi-Kebria, M. (2005). The results of two-stage surgical management of Hirschsprung's disease in a 10-Year Period. Retrieved November, 1, 2005, from the Department of Pediatric Surgery, Mofid Children's Hospital, Shahid Beheshti University of Medical Sciences website: http://www.ams.ac.ir

Klein, B., Philippart, A., (1993.) Hirschsprung's disease: three decades experience at a single institution. *Journal of Pediatric Surgery, 29*, 1291-1294.

Kleinhaus, S., Boley, S., Sheran, M. et al. (1979). Hirschsprung's disease. A survey of the members of the surgical section of the American Academy of Pediatrics. *Journal of Pediatric Surgery, 14*, 588-597.

Langer, J., Birnbaum, E., (1997). Preliminary experience with intrasphincteric botulinum toxin for persistent constipation after pull-through for Hirschsprung's disease. *Journal of Pediatric Surgery, 32*, 1059-1061.

Langer, J. (2002). Disorders of defecation in children: what is the role of the surgeon. *Digestive Health Matters*, Spring IFFGD 2002.

Larson, D. (1990). *Mayo Clinic Family Health Book.* New York: William Morrow and Co.

Laurence, K., Prosser, R., Rocker, I., Pearson, J., Richard, C. (1975). *Hirschsprung's disease associated with congenital heart malformation, broad big toes, and ulnar polydactyly in sibs: a case for fetoscopy.* Retrieved November 20, 2005, from http://jmg.bmjjournals.com

Laxatives. Retrieved April 3, 2007, from University of Michigan, Pediatric Surgery web site: http://pediatric.um-surgery.org

Laxatives. (n.d.). Retrieved April 3, 2007, from http://www.cancerhelp.org.uk

Leshin, L. MD. (1997). *Trisomy 21: The story of Down syndrome.* Retrieved November 19, 2005, from http://www.ds-health.com

Levitt, M., Falcone, R., Pena, A. (2007). Pediatric fecal incontinence, in: fecal incontinence: diagnosis and treatment. *Springer*, 341-350.

Levin, S., (1987). The immune system and susceptibility to infections in Down's syndrome. *Journal of Pediatric Surgery, 29,* 781.

Levitt, M., Pena, A. (2007). Follow-up and management of children operated on for an Anorectal malformation. Retrieved February, 19, 2007, from the Colorectal Center for Children, Cincinnati, Ohio. http://wwwcininattichildrens.org

Lewis, SJ., Heaton, KW (1997). Stool form scale as a useful guide to intestinal transit time. *Scand. J. Gastroenterol.* 32 (9): 920–4. doi:10.3109/00365529709011203. PMID 9299672.

Longworth, L., Young T., Beath S., et.al (2006). An economic evaluation of pediatric small bowel transplantation in the United Kingdom. *Transplantation, 82,* 508-515.

Ludman, L., Spitz, L., Tsuji, H., Pierro, A. (2002). Hirschsprung's disease: functional and psychological follow up comparing total colonic and rectosigmoid aganglionosis. *Archives of Disease in Childhood, 86,* 348-351.

Majamaa, H., Isolauri, E. (1997). Probiotics: A novel approach in the management of food allergy. *Journal of Allergy clin. 99 (2),* 179-185.

Marker of Disease. (n.d.). Retrieved November 19, 2005, from http://www.bamc.amedd.army.mil

Mayo Clinic. (2005). Children and constipation: ways to cope and when to worry. Retrieved April 23, 2005, from http://www.mayoclinic.com

Mayo Clinic. (2007). Diaper Rash. Retrieved February 22, 2007, from http://www.mayoclinic.com

Mayo Clinic. (2005). The lowdown on laxatives: know your options. Retrieved April 23, 2005, from http://www.mayoclinic.com

McCallion, A., Stames, E., Conlon, R., Aravidna. (2003). *Phenotype variation in two -locus mouse models of Hirschsprung tissue-specific interaction between RET and EDNRB.* Retrieved October 24, 2005, from http://www.pubmedcentral.gov

Medcyclopedia. Hirschsprung's Disease. (n.d.). Retrieved March 10, 2005 from http:www.amershamhealth.com

Medical Encyclopedia: Riley-Day syndrome. (n.d.). Retrieved November 18, 2005, from http://www.hlm.nih.gov

MEN 2. (n.d.) Retrieved November 19, 2005, from http://www.orpha.net

MEN Syndromes. (n.d.) Retrieved November 19, 2005, from http://www.thedoctorsdoctor.com

Merck Manual Home Edition. (2007). Candidiasis: fungal skin infections. Retrieved February 2, 2007, from http://www.merck.com

Mital, B., Garg, S. (1995). Anticarcinogenic, hypocholeterolemic and antagonistic activities of Lactobacillus acidophilus. *Crit Rev Microbiol, 21,* 175-214.

Moore, B., Singaram C., Eckhoff, D., Gaumnite, E., Starling, J. (1996).

Immunohistochemical evaluations of ultrashort-segment Hirschsprung's Disease. *Journal of Pediatric Surgery, 39,* 817-822.

Morrison, S. (2003). *Stem cell defects are key to Hirschsprung's Disease, say U-M scientists.* Retrieved May 31, 2005 from University of Michigan Medical School Web Site: http://www.med.umich.edu

Multiple Endocrine Neoplasia, Type 2. (n.d.). Retrieved November, 19, 2005, from http://www.orpha.net

Multiple Congenital Anomaly/Mental Retardation (MCA/MR) syndromes. (n.d.). Retrieved November 20, 2005, from http://www.nlm.nih.gov

National Digestive Diseases Information Clearinghouse (NDDIC). (2001). What I need to know about Hirschsprung's disease. Retrieved November 8, 2003, from http://digestive.niddk.nih.gov

Nixon, H. (1985). *A color atlas of surgery for Hirschsprung's disease.* Netherlands: Wolfe Medical Publications Ltd.

Ondine's Curse. (n.d.) Retrieved November 18, 2005, from http://www.answers.com

Parenting. (2007). Treating diaper rash. Retrieved February 24, 2007, from http://health.yahoo.com

Parker, J., Philip M. (2002). *The official Parent's Sourcebook on Hirschsprung's Disease*. San Diego: ICON Health Publications

Pavan, W. (1998) NIH scientists identify new Hirschsprung's disease gene. Retrieved January 5, from http://www.genome.gov

Pavan, W. (2005). Hirschsprung's disease. The National Human Genome Institute. Retrieved March 30, from http://www.genome.gov

Pfefferkorn, M., Croffie, J., Corkins, M., Gupta, S., Fitzgerald, J. (2003). Impact of sedation and anesthesia on the rectoanal inhibitory reflex in children. *JPGN, 38*, 324-327.

Pheochromocytoma. (n.d.) Retrieved September 18, 2005, from http://www.fpnotbook.com

Pheochromocytoma. (n.d.) Retrieved November 19, 2005, from http://www.endocrineweb.com

Pobojewski, S., Morrison, S. (2003) Stem cell defects are key to Hirschsprung's disease, say U-M Scientists. Retrieved August 14, from http://www.med.umich.edu

Proctology.us. (2005) Hirschsprung's disease. Retrieved April 21, from http://www.proctology.us/hd.php

Quick Study: A weekly digest of new research on major health topics/ constipation. (2006, August 22). *Washington Post*. Retrieved from http://www.washingtonpost.com

Quinn, F., Surana, R., Puri, P. (1994). The influence of trisomy 21 on outcome in children with Hirschsprung's Disease. *Journal of Pediatric Surgery, 29,* 781.

Rintala, R., Landahl, H. (2001). Sodium cromoglycate in the management of chronic or recurrent enterocolitis in patients with Hirschsprung's disease. *Journal of Pediatric Surgery, 36,* 1032-1035.

Rocky Mountain Pediatric Surgery. (2005). Patient care- Hirschsprung's disease colonic aganglionosis. Retrieved July 7, from http://www.pediatricsurgeon.com

Rotavirus. (n.d.). Retrieved July 14, 2007, from http://www.rotavirusinfo.com

Ruysch, F., Observationum anatomico-chirugicarum centuria. *Obs, 92,* 118. Henricum et viduram Theodri Boom. Amstelodum, 1691.

Sawin, B. (2005). Surgeon in Chief. Seattle Children's Hospital. Seattlechildrens.org

Saxton, M., Ein, S., Hoehner, J., Kim, P. (2000). Near-total intestinal aganglionosis: Long-term follow-up of a morbid condition. *Journal of Pediatric Surgery, 35,* 669-672.

Schmieden, V. (1913). Retrospect of Surgery: The operative treatment of persistent Constipation. *Canadian Medical Association Journal, 4,* 69-70.

Seigel-Maier, L. (1999, January). Pro-digestion with probiotics. *Better Nutrition. (n.p.).*

Shen, L., Pichel, J., Mayeli, T., Sariola, H., Westphal, H. (2002). *Gdnf haploinsufficiency causes Hirschsprung-like intestinal obstruction and early-onset lethality in mice.* Retrieved October 24, from http://www.pubmedcentral.gov

Spence, A (1986). *Basic human anatomy, second edition.* Menlo Park: Benjamin/Cummings Publishing Company, Inc.

Swenson, O. (1949). New concepts of the etiology, diagnosis, and treatment of congenital megacolon (Hirschsprung's disease). *American Academy of Pediatrics. 4,* 201-209.

Symptoms of enteroviruses. (n.d.). Retrieved January 5, 2006, from http://www.wrongdiagnosis.com

Teitlelbaum, D., Coran, C., Weitzman, J. (1998). Hirschsprung's disease and related neuromuscular disorders of the intestines. In O'Neil JA Jr., Rowe Mi, Grosfeld, JL, et al. *Pediatric Surgery. 5th ed. (pp. 1381-424).* St. Louis, MO: Mosby-Yearbook.

Teitelbaum, D., Qualman, S., Caniano, D. (1988) Hirschsprung's disease. Identification of risk factors for enterocolitis. *Annals of Surgery, 207,* 240.

Testa, G., Holterman, M., Abcarian, H., Iqbal, R., Benedetti, E. (2008). Simultaneous or sequential combined living donor-intestine transplantation in children. *Transplantation, 85(5),* 713-715.

That little voice in your stomach. (n.d.) Retrieved November, 11, 2005, from http://whyfiles.org

The Cleveland Clinic Health Information Center. (2005). Laparoscopic intestinal surgery: a guide for patients. Retrieved October 21, 2005, from http://www.clevelandclinic.org

The Oley Foundation (1996). Septic complications of TPN. Retrieved September 30, 2005, from http://www.oley.org

Thomas, D., Fernie, D., Bayston, R., Spitz, L, Nixon, H. (1986). Enterocolitis in Hirschsprung's disease: a controlled study of the etiologic role of Clostridium difficile. *Journal of Pediatric Surgery, 21(1),* 22-25.

Tomita, R., Munakata, K., Fukuzawa, M. (2000). Pathogenesis and management of the chronic constipation in children. Electophysiological assessments of children with chronic constipation. *Japanese Journal of Pediatric Surgery, 32,* 251-258.

Turnock, R., Spitz, L., Strobel, S. (1992). A study of mucosal gut immunity in infants who develop Hirschsprung's –associated enterocolitis. *Journal of Pediatric Surgery, 27,* 828.

University of Michigan Section of Pediatric Surgery. (n.d.). Enterocolitis Associated with Hirschsprung's Disease. Retrieved May 26, 2005, from http://pediatric.um-surgery.org

Vanderwinden, J. (1999). Role of interstitial cells of cajal and their relationship with the enteric nervous system, *Eur J Morphol, 37 (4-5),* 250-256.

Van Kuyk, E., Brugman, A., Wissink, M., Oerlemans, H., Severijnen, R., Bleijenberg, G. (2001). Defecation problems in children with Hirschsprung's disease: a prospective controlled study of a multi-disciplinary behavioral treatment. *Acta Paediatr, 90,* 1153-1159.

Waardenburg syndrome. (n.d.) Retrieved November 18, 2005, from the University of Maryland Medical Center Web site: http://www. umm.edu

Weale, A., Edwards, A., Bailey, M., Lear, P. (2005). Intestinal adaptation after massive intestinal resection. *Postgraduate Medical Journal, 81,* 178-184.

Wester, T. (1999). *Aspects of the human enteric nervous system.* Sweden: Eklundhofs Grafiska, AB.

What is Neuroblastoma? (n.d.). Retrieved October 21, 2005, from http://www.cancer.org.

Wikipedia Encyclopedia. Hirschsprung's Disease. (n.d.). Retrieved January 18, 2005, http://en.widipedia.org/wiki/Hirschsprung's_disease

Wikipedia Encyclopedia. Ondine's Curse. (n.d.). Retrieved January 5, 2005, from http://en.wikipedia.org

Wikipedia Encyclopedia. Total Parenteral Nutrition. (n.d.). Retrieved July 8, 2008, from http://en.wikipedia.org

Wilcox, D., Bruce, J., Bowen, J., Bianchi, A., Neblett, W. (1997). One-stage neonatal pull-through to treat Hirschsprung's Disease. *Journal of Pediatric Surgery, 32,* 243-247.

Wilson-Storey, D., Scobie, W.G. (1989). Impaired gastrointestinal mucosal defense in Hirschsprung's disease: a clue to the pathogenesis of enterocolitis? *Journal of Pediatric Surgery, 24,* 462.

Witsell, D., Garrett C., Yarbrough, W., Dorrestein, S., Drake, A., Weissler, M. (1995). Effect of Lactobacillus acidophilus on antibiotic-associated gastrointestinal morbidity: a prospective randomized trial. *J. Otolaryngol, 24 (4),* 230-233.

Wood, J. (2008). Enteric nervous system: reflexes pattern generators and motility. *Animal Genetics, 39,* 51-61.

World of Science. Chromosome, Gene and DNA. (n.d.). Retrieved November 23, 2005, from http://www.vigyanprasar.com

Yamatake, A., Kato, Y., Tibboel, D., Murata, Y., Sueyoshi, N., Fujimoto, T., Nishiye, H., Miyano, T. (1995). *A lack of intestinal pacemaker (c-kit) in aganglionic bowel of patients with Hirschsprung's disease.* Retrieved November 11, 2005, from http://www.ncbi.nlm.hih.gov

Ziegler, M., Royal, R., Brandt, J., Drasnin, J., Martin, L. (1993). Extended myectomy-myotomy. A therapeutic alternative for total intestinal aganglionosis. *Annals of Surgery, 218,* 504-511.

INDEX

undescended testicles, 132
urogenital echographic, 133
urostomy bag, 114

V

voluntary nervous system, 25
Vomiting, 26, 65
v-shaped mouth, 128

W

washouts, 67
weight loss, 134
Wilhelm Johannsen, 91
witch hazel, 78

X

x-rays, 35

Y

yeast rash, 62

Z

Zinc oxide, 63
Zofran™, 105

www.ingramcontent.com/pod-product-compliance
Lightning Source LLC
Chambersburg PA
CBHW020706270326
41928CB00005B/286